KETO DIET OVER 50

Ketogenic Diet for Senior Beginners & Weight Loss Book After 50.
Reset Your Metabolism with this
Complete Guide for Women
+ 2 Weeks Meal Plan

Dr. Gillian Keys Pomroy, Dr. Anna Bernardi

CONTENTS

Introduction

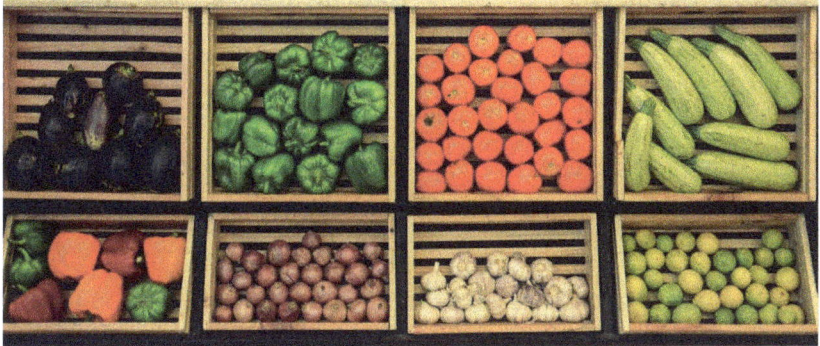

This is a beginner's guide to successfully maintaining a Keto diet, as a woman over the age of 50-years-old. Over the last few years, you have likely heard a lot about the Keto diet. It is known as being a diet that allows you to indulge, while still promoting weight loss. People of all ages have seen its incredible benefits.

Packed with foods that are rich in protein and high in fat and doing away with carbohydrates is the ultimate way that the Keto diet helps you to lose weight and maintain a healthy body. Instead of burning carbs, your body will be trained to burn fats, boosting your metabolism in an efficient way. It also turns your fats into ketones in your liver, which ends up providing you with additional energy for your brain.

Instead of focusing on the carbs that you will be giving up, the Keto diet aims its focus on all of the protein and fats that your body craves. Imaginably, there are many delicious recipes that you can follow and foods that you can eat, even when you aren't at home. The Keto diet is known for being one of the least restrictive diets; an important aspect in helping you to follow through with it. This guide will answer all of the questions that you have about what the diet consists of and how to successfully make Keto a part of your daily life. Unlike other diets, you will be amazed at how much freedom you are still allowed. It is almost like you aren't even on a diet at all!

As your body and brain ages, it is important to pay attention to all of the ways in which you can successfully maintain your energy levels. Certain tasks become a lot more cumbersome when you are running on half the energy than you're used to. The Keto diet works very well for women, especially those over 50. Aside from the benefits to your metabolism and energy levels, you will also notice a decrease in inflammation, a stable blood sugar level, and balanced hormones. With all of these benefits in place, you will notice that you will feel better both physically and mentally. And, of course, your mental health is very important to consider while on a diet. A lot of diets cause you to feel that you are lacking what you truly want to eat, therefore putting you into a negative mindset.

Keto is different and this guide will show you all of the reasons why. It is an overall lifestyle change that is possible for almost everyone, no matter what your average day looks like. You will be filled with plenty of optimism and all of the positivity necessary in order to meet your goals. Whether you want to maintain your current weight or lose weight in the process, Keto will help you get to where you truly want to be. It will become an anti-aging diet that will ultimately be a regular part of your everyday life.

You will experience all of these wonderful benefits as you begin your own Keto journey:

- Weight loss that lasts

- Lower blood sugar levels

- More energy

- Younger looking skin

- A boosted metabolism

- Balanced hormones

- Anti-aging benefits that work from the inside out

- A wide variety of delicious meals to eat

Most women can get the hang of Keto right away and experience few difficulties maintaining the diet. With the assistance of this guide, all of your questions about Keto will be fully answered.

If you are ready to feel great and look great, then you are ready to begin your own Keto diet. It will be a diet like no other because you will feel great every step of the way. There are no tricks or deceiving steps that you must take in order to succeed with the diet. As long as you are educated on what you need to be eating, you should have no problem incorporating the Keto diet into your current lifestyle. So, let's jump in and learn about the Keto diet, and how it can help you!

CHAPTER 1

The History of the Ketogenic Diet: What is Keto?

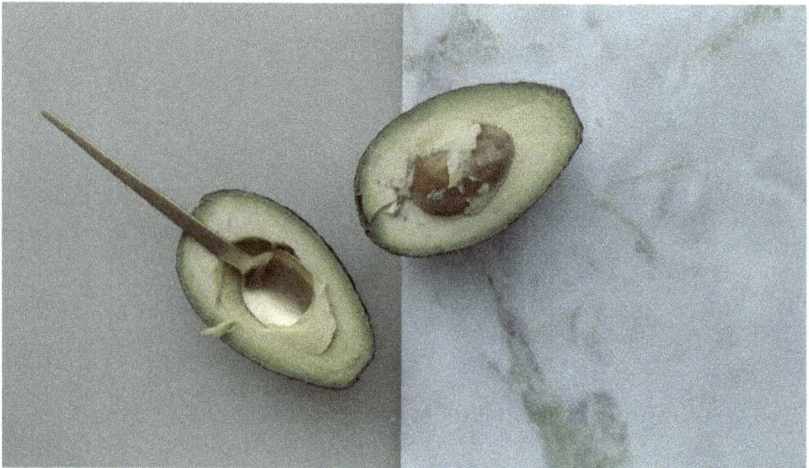

The Keto diet follows one basic principle — eliminate simple carbs and eat more fats in order to keep your body in a state of "fasting." When your body gets into this state, it will begin to burn ketones instead of burning glucose. Overall, this is thought to make you healthier without having to limit the quantity of food that you are eating on a daily basis.

Basically, the diet follows a model of 60-75% healthy fat consumption, 15-30% protein consumption, and only 5-10% carbs consumption, in order to change the way that you process energy. A lot of people are skeptical at first because it seems like it is a diet with minimal rules; but it truly is that simple.

Putting your body into a state of ketosis is ultimately your main goal. Your system normally chooses to run on glucose, which is sugar. When you eliminate the consumption of carbs, this causes your body to think that it is "starving," but you won't feel that way. From this point, your body will make the necessary adjustments that it needs to make in order to shift its focus. It will then generate a secondary source of energy that is derived from fat in order to keep the glucose flowing to the brain. Without the presence of so many carbs, your body will break down all of the fat compounds into ketones; an alternative fuel source.

Many people have realized that following this diet provides impressive results. Not only will your weight be properly managed, but you will also end up feeling healthier and more energized than ever before. The term "ketogenic" is fairly new, only being used since the 20th century. But even before this term was introduced, the Ancient Greeks were big advocates for restricting diets in order to treat diseases such as epilepsy. An interesting history, indeed, that deserves a quick exploration.

Back in the days of Hippocrates, fasting was the only known treatment for epilepsy. This became a very standard practice over the next two thousand years. It began to spread from Europe throughout the whole world. While today, most people utilize the Keto diet to manage their weight and health, its origins very clearly state that it was meant to reprogram the brain. Epileptic patients in 1911 were recorded having fewer seizures and fewer epilepsy symptoms while on a Keto diet versus being on a regular diet. It only took a few periods of regular fasting for them to see these results.

It was around the same time in the United States that an osteopathic physician, Hugh Conklin, started to recommend fasting as a treatment method for his epileptic patients. They would fast for 18-25 days at a time, and the success rates were incredible. Most patients reported that they experienced a 50% success rate, for adults, and a whopping 90% success rate for children. Of course, this is an extreme version of the now-refined diet that we know about today. While the results were very impressive, health professionals knew that this wasn't a permanent solution. Fasting is inherently temporary. Once the patients returned to their normal diets, the seizures would come back just as quickly.

Once this problem became apparent, doctors got to work in order to modify the treatment plan into one that could become long-lasting. Instead of restricting all calories equally, doctors began focusing on eliminating only certain sugars and starches to study these effects. Dr. Wilder at the Mayo Clinic was a well-known physician who took part in the studies. He noticed right away that his patients were having fewer seizures with their lower blood sugar levels. Dr. Wilder was responsible for officially creating the Keto diet as a lifestyle instead of merely a temporary treatment plan. The diet that we are all familiar with now mimics the way that your metabolism reacts during a period of fasting.

A simple concept evolved into a simple diet plan. Patients were able to stay in a permanent state of fasting without actually feeling that they were starving themselves. This shift in what you consume triggers your body to automatically receive the benefits of the ketones. This allowed people to feel that they were still getting all of the calories and nutrition that they needed but tricked the body into metabolizing as if they were starving. It was a fascinating discovery that truly shaped the Keto diet into what it is today.

Another Mayo Clinic physician, Dr. M.G. Peterman was credited for standardizing the diet. He called it the "classic keto" approach. This is an approach that is often still used today. A 4:1 ratio of fat to protein and carbs must be maintained. 90% of all calories come from fat, while 6% come from protein and only 4% from carbs. This is often thought of as an ideal approach to the Keto diet, while a 3:1 ratio is also considered highly beneficial. This might sound extreme on paper, but it truly isn't hard to maintain because your body still recognizes that it is getting all of the nutrition that it needs.

There is typically one big question that remains after reading about the Keto diet, and that involves what you can actually eat. Historically, the following foods were known as essentials while being on the diet:

- Vegetables without Starch: broccoli, cauliflower, cabbage, leafy greens, onions, and peppers

- Full Fat Dairy: Cheese, yogurt, and milk

- Protein: eggs, soybeans, shellfish, fish, pork, poultry, and beef

- Nuts and Seeds: almonds, pistachios, walnuts, sunflower seeds, and pumpkin seeds

- Quality Fats: unlimited from both plant and animal sources

- Fruits (sparingly): avocado, rhubarb, coconut, and berries

Doctors would put emphasis on using precise measurements in order to achieve the maximum results. These ratios would be followed very carefully. It became so precise that the food was measured to the gram before each patient was able to consume it. The medical professionals could now see that this diet that mimicked fasting could be maintained for far longer periods of time.

Now, two centuries later the Keto diet has remained fairly unchanged. Nutritionists have created guidelines that suggest participants consume one gram of protein per kilogram of body weight. 10-15 grams of carbohydrates are acceptable, with the rest of the diet being focused on eating fats.

Scientifically, it is still hard to explain why the Keto diet is and was so successful for epileptics. The main theory that has been created states that the ketones' natural structures cause them to have an anti-electrical response in the brain. This means that people who experience seizures are no longer being exposed to these electrical currents, therefore preventing future seizures from occurring. It is fascinating to think about its results regarding epileptic patients, but the benefits are not limited. It didn't take much time for doctors to realize that the Keto diet could also benefit those who were not epileptic.

Interestingly enough, this discovery came when the diet was tested on children. The children who were put on the diet were noted as being less irritable, more focused, and easier to discipline. They were also to get better sleep at night, further benefiting them. Follow up research has since been done in the 2000s and it showed the same results. With the development of anticonvulsant drugs, the eating strategy was pushed aside. The Keto diet only recently resurfaced as a valid diet plan and lifestyle choice.

During this time when the Keto approach was being set aside, it lost a lot of momentum. This caused people to use it incorrectly, not following its precise measurements. Fewer dieticians were experienced with the diet and did not know how to properly coach their patients through it. Because of these bad experiences, people saw the Keto diet as something negative and ineffective. In just a matter of decades, the Keto diet had a bad stigma attached to it that prevented people from wanting to experience it. This marked a time period of the initial disappearance of the Keto diet, used as a treatment plan or diet plan.

Revisiting Keto

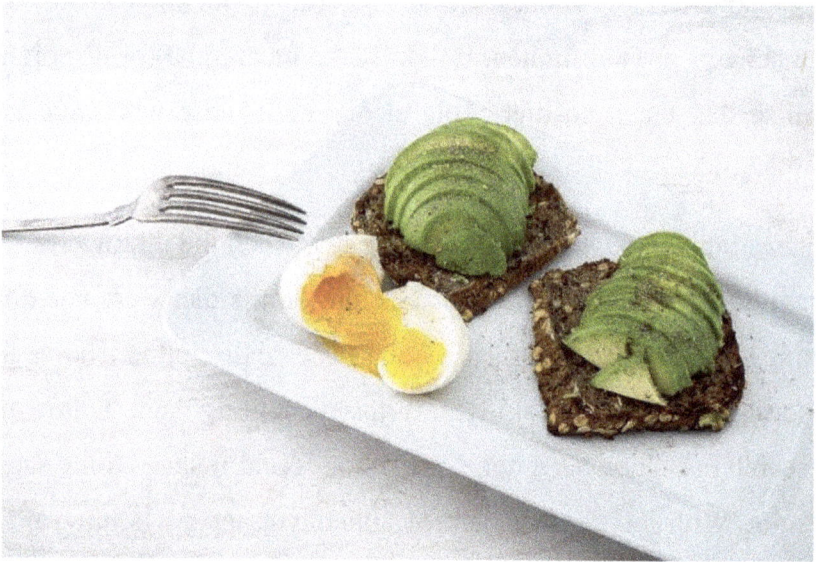

Keto returned to the mainstream in the 1990s. Those who were still interested in it studied it because of its mysterious workings rather than as a diet plan to follow. This went on for the next several years until an episode of the news television program Dateline, in 1994, shed some positive light on Keto.

In the episode, a 2-year-old child was featured. He had been experiencing severe epilepsy. His seizures were out of control until he was placed on the Keto diet. It was a risky move, but his doctors at John Hopkins did not know what else to try. The severity of his disorder led them down the Keto path. At this time, fewer than 10 children were being treated in this way for epilepsy each year.

After the show aired, it triggered a major response from medical professionals and regular people alike. Not to mention, a huge increase in scientific interest. All of the gears began turning again as people took interest in the Keto diet once again. It even led to the creation of a film called "First Do No Harm," created by this child's father. Released in 1997, the movie starred Meryl Streep and revolves around the experience of with the diet and how much it helped their child. It aired on national television, creating even more of a buzz around the topic.

This renewed interest in Keto led us to the modern-day experience of the diet that we are most familiar with. Hospitals began offering it as a reliable treatment plan once again. Epilepsy was now being treated as it had been in the past when the Keto diet was first established. To this day, the Keto diet is used as a treatment plan in nearly all major children's hospitals. It continually attracts interest from scientists and other medical professionals because of its role in the treatment of neurological disorders. However, the story does not end there.

If the Keto diet were only beneficial to those who were experiencing epilepsy, its interest may have died down by now. Since the diet has been back in the spotlight, a lot of people have realized how beneficial it is for controlling physical health and weight management. Once this perspective of the Keto diet shifted, it gained a lot of attention from those wishing to live a healthier lifestyle. This renewed interest in Keto allowed researchers to see that it could be used as solely a diet plan, even for those who were completely neurologically healthy.

It took additional time for Keto to really become a trustworthy diet plan that is used by people who do not have epilepsy. While it was regaining momentum in the 90s, so was the Atkins diet. If you have been following diet trends for the last few decades, you likely already know what Atkins entails. This diet plan has a similar outlook when it comes to carbs and the way it was presented really took off during this time. Though Atkins dominated the spotlight, this allowed even more room for scientists and researchers to take Keto seriously as a standalone diet plan. The two were compared to each other often in the late 90s, making room for the diet that we now know so much about.

In today's society, Atkins has slowly faded away to make room for Keto. A lot of people found Atkins to be too strict and complicated. Eating out or away from home was a challenge for those partaking in the diet plan. Keto aimed to change this perspective. It proved to people that they can still lose weight and maintain a satisfying lifestyle while doing so. Many would argue that being on Keto does not feel like a diet plan at all. Instead, it acts as a guideline for how we need to treat our bodies by providing a method that is simple yet effective. Keto is so enjoyable because it doesn't ask you to count calories every single day. It is a more flexible diet plan that allows individuals to still feel that they are individuals.

Aside from proving itself to nutritionists and people alike, Keto is thriving in a time where social media is very popular. As people go through their Keto journeys, it is easy to access this real-time progress in a way that feels comforting and informative. On any given social media platform, it is not usual to see that people are posting about their experience with the Keto diet. Along with this praise, people also love to post pictures of their food! While the early 2000s gave us a lot more freedom of information thanks to the internet, this current decade allows us to dive even deeper. Seeing these real experiences that people are having with Keto makes it more relatable. It also gives us ideas for recipes and how the Keto diet can be enjoyed.

The message remains simple to this day — pay attention to how your body feels. Starting any new diet plan can be questionable, especially if you do not know exactly how to execute it and apply it to your own life. The findings behind the Keto diet continue to impress those of varying backgrounds and in different geographical locations. When first starting your own Keto journey, your body is going to feel different immediately. This is because of what is actually going on internally. Unlike many other gimmick diets or fads, Keto doesn't promise rapid or unrealistic weight loss. Instead, it provides an overall lifestyle solution that can be followed by anyone.

Whether you are still on the fence about starting your own Keto journey or you have all of the resources that you need, the results will speak for themselves. Naturally, our bodies weaken as we age. This can send us into a frenzy of trying the latest health crazes and forcing us to eat foods that we don't really enjoy. Being open-minded about Keto is important in the beginning. As long as you are listening to your body, keeping your portions similar to what you are used to eating, and being creative with your meals, you will find that the Keto journey can be a wonderful addition to your life.

As a woman over 50, you have an awareness about your overall health that you probably didn't have when you were younger. And, that's natural. The purpose of this book is to help you bring that awareness into action - specifically tapping into the benefits of the Keto diet. While it's a relatively easy change to make in your life, there are things you need to know before you dive in, that we'll be covering throughout this book. First and foremost, the different types and strategies of ketogenic diets. So, we'll start there next.

CHAPTER 2

Types of Ketogenic: SKD, TKD, and CKD

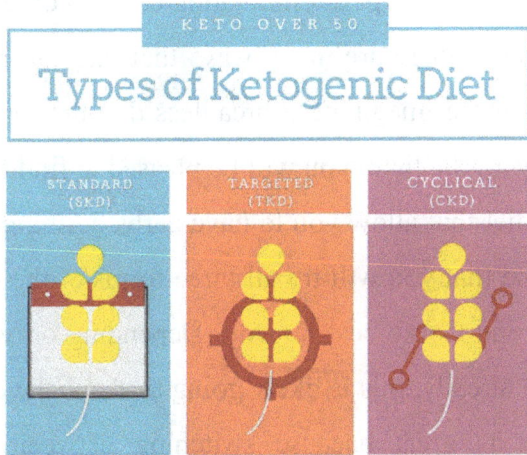

Having flexibility with your diet plan is a significant positive factor in being able to stick with it. While you now have a basic understanding of how Keto came to be, there is also more information to delve into by researching the various types of the diet that you can follow. If you do not want to take a standard approach, know that you do have options.

Keto actually allows you to modify the diet in three different ways depending on what you currently need. This gives you even more freedom to feel great and to feel like you are not on a diet at all. Most other diet plans do not have these options, making them seem stricter. Keto aims to give everyone a plan that works for them, not just a single template that must be followed.

The difference between these forms of Keto comes in the percentages of the foods that you will be eating. While they all believe in the core concept of eliminating carbs in order to get your body into ketosis, there are many ways that this can be done. For example, if you are imagining a breadless diet that will leave you feeling cranky all the time, you will be pleased to find that there are forms of the diet that allow you to have carbs during certain times. You might find that you will try all three forms of the diet in order to see which one works best for you. Depending on what you are used to eating already, this is likely going to shape the decision that you make. It is great because switching between these three variations is not extreme or dangerous. They vary just enough to give you options without sacrificing your health in the process.

SKD: Standard Keto Diet

The standard Keto diet is likely the one that you have heard about the most. It is the plan that people generally like to start with because it provides a great foundation and introduction to the lifestyle. This diet involves a low-carb and moderate-protein approach. The focus is on maintaining a high-fat meal plan.

An example of the SKD includes the individual eating 75% fat, 20% protein, and 5% carbs. (This is the general guideline that you will follow each day.) People enjoy this method because it does not change; these simple principles are relatively easy to maintain once you get used to them. The SKD has been studied the most extensively. When you read about Keto, it is likely the SKD method that researchers are referring to.

A summary of its benefits includes effective weight loss. For most, this is one of the biggest concerns when starting any diet plan. If you feel that you want to lose weight safely, the SKD will allow you to do so in a healthy way. The reason why this works so well is that you never experience periods of intense hunger like you would with other diets. At no point in time should you feel that you are truly starving yourself when you are on the Keto diet. This feeling will only lead to negative results because the body will want to stray from the plan. You've probably experienced this first-hand while trying other diets. When you are hungry enough, you lose motivation and are more prone to eat unhealthy foods that tend to "comfort" you. Losing progress in this way can become very discouraging.

Another benefit of being on the SKD is that your risk factor for diseases and ailments will be lowered. Giving you a well-rounded meal plan, Keto aims to push you in a healthy direction that you can easily take. Because you won't be consumed with counting calories or limiting your food intake, you will be able to fully appreciate this benefit while you are on the diet. Keto feels so great because it is a lot different than a low-fat diet. Since your body is still getting plenty of protein, you will be less likely to stray. One study has actually found that being on the Keto diet has shown a success rate with weight loss that is up to 2.2 times more effective than other similar diets.

Your risk factor for diabetes should be taken into account when starting the Keto diet. As you age, this risk factor can naturally increase. Two of the biggest problems have to do with a change in metabolism and a spike in your blood sugar. As you know, the SKD places a lot of focus on redirecting your metabolism and keeping your blood sugar down. While being on the Keto diet, you are going to be losing weight due to your body burning the bad fats that aren't necessary to its functionality. In turn, it will be getting rid of the excess fats that you do not need. This is another way that Keto can greatly benefit someone who is pre-diabetic or has a genetic history of diabetes.

The benefits do not end there. The SKD has been known for reducing your risk of cancer, heart disease, Alzheimer's, and polycystic ovary syndrome. With aging comes increased risks in many or all of these conditions. It is impressive to think that Keto can provide comprehensive benefits; enough to protect you from all of these diseases. By not giving up all of the foods that you love, you will feel great about your journey.

Keeping in mind that Keto is not only effective but preventative, may increase your motivation as you plan out your meals and figure out what other aspects of your life must be changed in order to adjust the way you are eating. It isn't hard to remember what to do while on Keto. As long as you are staying away from sugary foods, both natural and artificial, you are allowing your body to adjust to the diet naturally. Placing a focus on making meat and dairy taste delicious, you won't even notice the carbs that you are replacing.

TKD: Targeted Keto Diet

The targeted Keto diet focuses on workout plans that you have in place. While you know that sticking to a healthy diet is very important, another aspect of this is your effort placed on exercising and getting up and moving. The main difference between the TKD and the SKD is that you will actually be consuming carbs before you work out. This will provide you with a boost of energy when you need it most, allowing you to focus on your physical fitness. The amount of exercise that you are doing needs to increase and be modified as you age. You likely can't do the things that you used to do when you were younger, but that doesn't mean that physical fitness needs to be put in the background. Staying very much in the foreground, taking part in the TKD means that you need to have a solid fitness routine.

In order to make this plan work for you, it takes a little bit of preparation before you actually begin to change your eating habits. Think about the exercises that you enjoy doing and that are suitable for your current level of physical fitness. While there is always room for growth and an increase in intensity, you need to start with something basic in order to not overdo it. Starting with light to moderate exercise twice weekly, you will be able to begin building your diet around your fitness routine. The principle is simple — eat Keto for five days out of the week and then eat carbs on the two days that you intend on getting your exercise in. This plan is for those who intend on keeping up with a regular fitness routine. It will show you adverse effects if you eat based on the TKD method without including exercise in the plan.

You can still have a fat loss goal while following the TKD plan. What is essential to remember is that you do not overeat on your days of carb-consumption. Since you are going to be allowing your body carbs selectively, you need to remember that these carbs are going to count as calories. Because of this, you also need to adjust the number of fats that you are eating on those days. It all needs to balance itself out and this can be the trickiest part of getting the hang of the TKD. Only you can hold yourself accountable for how much exercise you plan on completing and how many carbs you plan on eating. It can take some trial and error to get this ratio right, but that is normal

The TKD is a middle ground between the SKD and the CKD. It allows you to perform at a high intensity for short periods of time without taking your body out of ketosis for too long. For many, the TKD has been shown to build up endurance and allow you to truly evolve with your physical fitness goals. This plan is most appropriate for those who are beginner-intermediate level with the Keto diet. If this sounds like something that can be incorporated into your lifestyle, you will find many benefits to this targeted approach. It allows you to aim higher with your fitness goals, showing you yet another reason how the Keto diet is not a diet filled with limitations or strictness.

Over time, exercise is going to feel less strenuous. When you get to this point, it is a good idea to revisit your fitness plan to see if it is still suitable for you. While it isn't great to change your diet frequently, you can safely adjust the TKD if you feel that you are ready to move up to more intense physical activity. Know that this is simply an option that it provides. You do not have to change anything if you feel that your body is doing well and that you are maintaining growth in your endurance. It is best to stick with your diet for at least a month before altering it too much. When you do consume your carbs, it is best to do so 30 minutes prior to exercising. Many people find that 25-50 grams of carbs are the right amount to allow them to power through their workouts.

CKD: Cyclical Keto Diet

As implied earlier, the CKD method is going to be the form of Keto that fluctuates the most. This diet plan involves a rotation that has you switching from the traditional high-fat, low-carb regimen to one that allows for higher carb intake. Of all the types of Keto, this one involves the most structure and guidelines. In the CKD, you are going to allow your body "refeeding days." This means that you will select a few days each week where you eat higher amounts of carbs in order to replenish your body's glucose levels. People choose to follow the CKD when they are focusing on muscle growth. Bodybuilders and those who are more serious about working out tend to follow this plan, for instance. Be aware, however, of all the types of Keto that are followed today, the CKD has the least amount of research to back it.

Many people confuse the CKD with carb cycling, but the two are different. When you are carb cycling, you follow a similar structure of cutting carbs on some days and then replenishing your body with carbs on the other days. The week is usually divided by 4-6 days of lower carb intake and 1-3 days of higher carb intake. One main difference between carb cycling and the CKD is that the former does not allow you to reach a state of ketosis. This means that you are not going to be getting all of the benefits that Keto has to offer.

This plan is likely going to be least applicable to you, but it is still important to learn about it, as it is still a viable form of Keto that many follows. Basically, on standard days, the individual must consume fewer than 50 grams of carbs each day. Healthy fats should make up approximately 75% of the diet. Some options include avocados, eggs, dairy products, nut butters, and fatty meats. Protein makes up about 15-20% of this diet. On refeeding days, you can consume carbs in a larger amount. Carbs will actually make up about 60-70% of your total calories, with protein making up 15-20% and fats 5-10%. As you can see, there is a big fluctuation between standard days and refeeding days.

A common misconception is that those on the CKD eat a lot of bread in order to get their carbs on refeeding days. But, that's not the typical, or healthy recommendation. Generally, the CKD method means that the extra carbs come from healthier sources, like sweet potatoes, butternut squash, brown rice, quinoa, oats, and other whole-grain foods. As you can see, there is still discipline required on those days, even despite the spike in carb intake. All of these carbs are very high in vitamins and nutrients. Foods and drinks that are sugary and artificial are still avoided because they simply lack any valuable nutrients. If you are not planning on pairing your diet with a relatively intense workout plan and routine, the CKD is likely not going to be the diet that works for you.

We also suggest that you incorporate some intermittent fasting when following the CKD. This means that, after your refeeding days, you fast for a few hours at a time. This will get you back to ketosis quicker. Your workouts should be done following your refeeding days to take full advantage of ketosis and to get into a prime condition for muscle growth. Those who wish to follow the diet for simple weight management or anti-aging will not get any additional benefits by following the CKD because it is simply an intensified version of Keto. However, you can benefit from CKD if you regularly partake in high-intensity workouts on a weekly basis or are planning on incorporating that level of activity in your life.

The main benefit of the CKD method is the potential for muscle growth and endurance-building abilities when it comes to sports or other athletic activities. One downside is that people often complain of constipation while on the CKD because of the fluctuating refeeding days. In order to combat this, it is important to watch your fiber intake, and make sure to hydrate accordingly. The CKD is a big commitment when it comes to dieting and it is advised that you try to maintain the SKD for several months, before you transition into the CKD.

Whichever plan you select, SKD, TKD or CKD, will depend on your current state of health as well as your health goals. The bottom line is that the Keto diet can work for people who have a wide variety of needs and aspirations. But, why is the Keto diet perfect for women over 50? Let's explore that, next.

CHAPTER 3

Why Women Over 50?

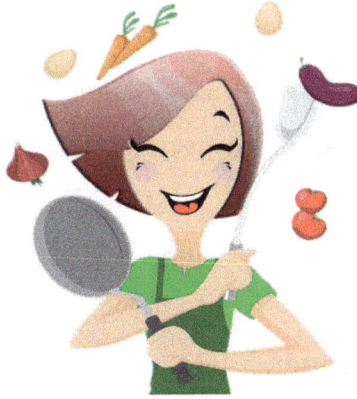

As a woman, you have likely experienced significant differences in the way that you must diet compared to the way that men can diet. Women tend to have a harder time losing weight because of their different hormones and the way their bodies break down fats. Another factor to consider is your age group. As the body ages, it is important to be more attentive with the way that you care for yourself. Aging bodies start to experience problems more quickly and this can be avoided with the proper diet and exercise plan. Keto works well for women of all ages and this is because of how it communicates with the body. No matter how fit you are right now or how much weight you need or want to lose, Keto is going to change the way that your body metabolizes, giving you a very personalized experience.

When starting your Keto diet, you should not be thinking about extremes because that isn't what Keto should be about. You should be able to place your body into ketosis without feeling terrible in the process. One of the biggest guidelines to follow while starting your Keto journey is that you need to listen to your body regularly. If you ever feel that you are starving or simply unfulfilled, then you will likely have to modify the way you are eating because it isn't reaching ketosis properly. It is not an overnight journey, so you need to remember to be patient with yourself and with your body. Adapting to a Keto diet takes a bit of transition time and a lot of awareness.

Why Keto for Women?

The health benefits of the Keto diet are not different for men or women, but the speed at which they are reached does differ. As mentioned, women's bodies are a lot different when it comes to the ways that they are able to burn fats and lose weight. For example, by design women have at least 10% more body fat than men. No matter how fit you are, this is just an aspect of being a woman that you must consider. Don't be hard on yourself if you notice that it seems like men can lose weight easier — that's because they can! What women have in additional body fat, men typically have the same in muscle mass. This is why men tend to see faster external results, because that added muscle mass means that their metabolism rates are higher. That increased metabolism means that fat and energy get burned faster. When you are on Keto, though, the internal change is happening right away.

Your metabolism is unique, but it is also going to be slower than a man's by nature. Since muscle is able to burn more calories than fat, the weight just seems to fall off of men, giving them the ability to reach the opportunity for muscle growth quickly. This should not be something that holds you back from starting your Keto journey. As long as you are keeping these realistic bodily factors in mind, you won't be left wondering why it is taking you a little bit longer to start losing weight. This point will come for you, but it will take a little bit more of a process that you must be committed to following through with.

Another unique condition that a woman can experience but a man cannot be PCOS or Polycystic Ovary Syndrome; a hormonal imbalance that causes the development of cysts. These cysts can cause pain, interfere with normal reproductive function, and, in extreme and dangerous cases, burst. PCOS is actually very common among women, affecting up to 10% of the entire female population. Surprisingly, most women are not even aware that they have the condition. Around 70% of women have PCOS that is undiagnosed. This condition can cause a significant hormonal imbalance, therefore affecting your metabolism. It can also inevitably lead to weight gain, making it even harder to see results while following diet plans. In order to stay on top of your health, you must make sure that you are going to the gynecologist regularly.

Menopause is another reality that must be faced by women, especially as we age. Most women begin the process of menopause in their mid-40s. Men do not go through menopause, so they are spared from yet another condition that causes slower metabolism and weight gain. When you start menopause, it is easy to gain weight and lose muscle. Most women, once menopause begins, lose muscle at a much faster rate, and conversely gain weight, despite dieting and exercise regimens. Keto can, therefore, be the right diet plan for you. Regardless of what your body is doing naturally, via processes like menopause, your internal systems are still going to be making the switch from running on carbs to deriving energy from fats.

When the body begins to successfully run on fats, you have an automatic fuel reserve waiting to be burned. It will take some time for your body to do this, but when it does, you will actually be able to eat fewer calories and still feel just as full because your body knows to take energy from the fat that you already have. This will become automatic. It is, however, a process that requires some patience, but being aware of what is actually going on with your body can help you stay motivated while on Keto.

Because a Keto diet reduces the amount of sugar you are consuming, it naturally lowers the amount of insulin in your bloodstream. This can actually have amazing effects on any existing PCOS and fertility issues, as well as menopausal symptoms and conditions like pre-diabetes and Type 2 diabetes. Once your body adjusts to a Keto diet, you are overcoming the things that are naturally in place that can be preventing you from losing weight and getting healthy. Even if you placed your body on a strict diet, if it isn't getting rid of sugars properly, you likely aren't going to see the same results that you will when you try Keto. This is a big reason why Keto can be so beneficial for women.

As we've discussed, carbs and sugar can have a huge impact on your hormonal balance. You might not even realize that your hormones are not in balance until you experience a lifestyle that limits carbs and eliminates sugars. Keto is going to reset this balance for you, keeping your hormones at healthy levels. As a result of this, you will probably find yourself in a better general mood, and with much more energy to get through your days.

For women over 50, there are guidelines to follow when you start your Keto diet. As long as you are following the method properly and listening to what your body truly needs, you should have no more problems than men do while following the plan. What you will have are more obstacles to overcome, but you can do it. Remember that plenty of women successfully follow a Keto diet and see great results. Use these women as inspiration for how you anticipate your own journey to go. On the days when it seems impossible, remember what you have working against you, but more importantly what you have working for you. Your body is designed to go into ketogenesis more than it is designed to store fat by overeating carbs. Use this as a motivation to keep pushing you ahead. Keto is a valid option for you and the results will prove this, especially if you are over the age of 50.

Why Keto for 50+?

As we age, we naturally look for ways to hold onto our youth and energy. It's not uncommon to think about things that promote anti-aging. Products and lifestyle changes are advertised everywhere, and they are designed to catch your attention, as you grapple with the reality of what it means to be a 50+ year-old woman in our society. Even if you aren't eating for the purposes of anti-aging yet, you have likely thought about it in terms of the way you treat your skin and hair, for example. The great thing about the Keto diet is that it supports maximum health, from the inside out; working hard to make sure that you are in the best shape that you can be in.

For instance, indigestion becomes common as you age. This happens because the body is not able to break down certain foods as well as it used to. With all of the additives and fillers, we all become used to putting our bodies through discomfort in an attempt to digest regular meals. You are probably not even aware that you are doing this to your body, but upon trying a Keto diet, you will realize how your digestion will begin to change. You will no longer feel bloated or uncomfortable after you eat. If you notice this as a common feeling, you are likely not eating food that is nutritious enough to satisfy your needs and is only resulting in excess calories.

Keto fills you up in all of the ways that you need, allowing your body to truly digest and metabolize all of the nutrients. When you eat your meals, you should not feel the need to overeat in order to overcompensate for not having enough nutrients. Anything that takes stress off of any system in your body is going to become a form of anti-aging. You will quickly find this benefit once you start your Keto journey, as it is one of the first-reported changes that most participants notice. In addition to a healthier digestive system, you will also experience more regular bathroom usage, with little to none of the problems often associated with age.

While weight loss is one of the more common desires for most 50+ women who start a diet plan, the way that the weight is lost matters. If you have ever shed a lot of weight before, you have probably experienced the adverse effects of sagging or drooping skin that you were left to deal with. Keto actually rejuvenates the elasticity in your skin. This means that you will be able to lose weight and your skin will be able to catch up. Instead of having to do copious amounts of exercise to firm up your skin, it should already be becoming firmer each day that you are on the Keto diet. This is something that a lot of participants are pleasantly surprised to find out.

Women also commonly report a natural reduction in wrinkles, and healthier skin and hair growth, in general. Many women who start the diet report that they actually notice reverse effects in their aging process. While the skin becomes healthier and more supple, it also becomes firmer. Even if you aren't presently losing weight, you will still be able to appreciate the effects that Keto brings to your skin and face. Because your internal systems are becoming healthier by the day, this tends to show on the outside in a short amount of time. You will also begin to feel healthier. While it is possible to read about the experiences of others, there is nothing like feeling this for yourself when you begin Keto.

Everyone, especially women over 50, has day-to-day tasks that are draining and require certain amounts of energy to complete. Aging can, unfortunately, take away from your energy reserve, even if you get enough sleep at night. It limits the way that you have to live your life, and this can become a very frustrating realization. Most diet plans bring about a sluggish feeling that you are simply supposed to get used to, for example. But Keto does the exact opposite. When you change your eating habits to fit the Keto guidelines, you are going to be hit with a boost of energy. Since your body is truly getting everything that it needs nutritionally, it will repay you with a sustained energy supply.

Another common complaint for women over 50 is that, seemingly overnight, your blood sugar levels are going to be more sensitive than usual. While it is important that everyone keeps an eye on these levels, it is especially important for those who are in their 50s and beyond. High blood sugar can be an indication that diabetes is on the way, but Keto can become a preventative measure, that we've already talked about. Additionally, naturally regulating elevated blood sugar levels, also reduces systemic inflammation, which is also common for women over 50. By balancing the immune system, of which inflammation is a part of, common aches and pains are reduced. If, for example, you've noticed that you have been feeling stiff lately, even despite your efforts to exercise and stretching, this is likely due to a normal case of inflamed joints. Inflammation can also affect vital organs and is a precursor to cancer. Keto will support your path to an anti-inflammatory lifestyle.

Sugar is never great for us, but it turns out that sugar can become especially dangerous as we age. What is known as a "sugar sag" can occur when you get older because the excess sugar molecules will attach themselves to skin and protein in your body. This doesn't even necessarily happen because you are eating too much sugar. Average levels of sugar intake can also lead to this sagging as the sugar weakens the strength of your proteins that are supposed to hold you together. With sagging comes even more wrinkles and arterial stiffening.

If you have any anti-aging concerns, the Keto diet will likely be able to address your worries. It is a diet that works extremely hard while allowing you a fairly simple and direct guideline to follow in return. While your motivation is necessary in order to form a successful relationship with Keto, you won't need to worry about doing anything "wrong" or accidentally breaking from your diet. As long as you know how to give up your sugary foods and drinks while making sure that you are consuming the correct amount of carbs, you will be able to find your own success while on the diet.

As a woman over 50, you'll find that you will feel better, healthier and younger, by implementing the simple steps that will tune your body into processing excess fats for energy. You'll build muscle, lose fat, and look and feel younger. As we've touched on, a Keto diet helps balance your hormones, reversing and/or eliminating many common menopausal signs and symptoms. Let's explore how, in the next chapter.

CHAPTER 4

Balance Hormones and Boost Energy

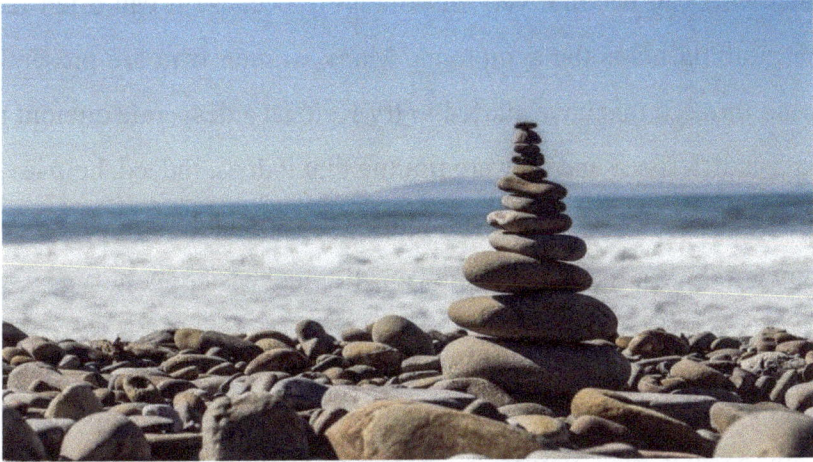

In the previous chapter, you learned a little bit about the ways in which Keto can provide great benefits for your hormones and energy levels. Considering how much you rely on both of these things each day, this is going to allow you to feel great while you are on the diet. There is nothing worse than starting a diet to find that it drags you down. Keto, when done correctly, will not make you feel this way. You will know that you are doing everything you need to do when you see that your energy is increasing. All of your hormones will also begin to balance out. This can leave you feeling naturally happier and calmer in your daily life.

If you have been experiencing difficulty with balancing your hormones, especially if you are going through menopause, you know how cumbersome these side effects can be. From hot flashes to mood swings, you have likely experienced it all in a very short period of time. This can become very discouraging because it can often feel that nothing helps the symptoms. Many women who are presently going through this have started to try Keto as a desperate attempt to make a difference and they are finding that it does, indeed, help level things out. Even if your symptoms are very bad, Keto has been shown to lessen them and make your life feel easier again.

It works so well because of the increase in fat consumption. While you have likely never been encouraged to consume *more* fat in any previous diet plan you've been on, Keto allows you to do this because it is literally changing the way that your body stores and breaks down this fat. When your body has more of these good fats inside, it will be prompted to create more estrogen and progesterone. This shows that, when you start a diet that slashes your fat consumption, you might actually be causing this hormonal imbalance to become more severe without even realizing it.

For those still dealing with periods, Keto helps by detoxifying the body. PMS symptoms are lessened when the body reaches this point of detoxification. PMS can become very hard to deal with because it produces an excess of estrogen. When you have too much estrogen in your system, this is when you will begin to feel cramping, bloating, and mood swings that you have been dealing with for years.

This estrogen dominance can occur more severely in certain cases when your diet consists of too many sugary foods. What you need is additional progesterone in order to balance you out. Because the Keto diet detoxifies you, it will be getting rid of the excess hormones that you don't need and begin to replace them with the ones that you are lacking.

As discussed, many women struggle with PCOS without even realizing it. While fertility might no longer be an issue for you, PCOS still brings forth many unpleasant side effects as you age. Because there is no cure for it, management of the disorder is essential. If you suffer from PCOS, poor blood sugar regulation and excess body fat can be making this a lot worse. Keto has been seen as a viable solution for easing the stress of PCOS. During a Duke University study, everyone who followed the diet found that they were able to lose weight and those seeking improvement with fertility were actually able to become healthy enough to get pregnant.

Insulin is a very big hormone that is important to your body. This controls your blood sugar and when this gets too low, can also begin to impact your sex hormone levels. What Keto does to your body is makes it more insulin sensitive. With a balanced level of insulin in your body, this will mean that your cells are going to use it properly. Studies have found that up to 75% of obese patients with diabetes experienced this positive increase in insulin sensitivity. An impressive number, these results appear very promising. While being more insulin sensitive, you are also able to get fit more easily.

Any weight you lose will be easier to keep off. This, in turn, lowers your risk for cardiovascular disease and dementia.

An instant way to feel depleted is by having to deal with copious amounts of stress with no relief. When you are handling the stressors in your daily life, your adrenal glands will begin to release cortisol in order to keep up with what is going on. This is your body's attempt at providing you with extra energy to handle the tough situations that you face. This can become a problem though, because your body can actually begin to produce too much cortisol. It also robs your body of the necessary estrogen and progesterone that it seeks.

While your body thinks that it is helping your stress by giving you this cortisol, it is actually detrimental to your sexual health, your muscle mass, and your overall point of burnout. The body is more fragile when it is in this heightened state and Keto aims to provide you with a more balanced approach. No one enjoys feeling like they just can't make it through their days, so it is best that you do not let your body overcompensate for what it mistakenly thinks that you need. The Keto diet will redirect it and guide you in the right direction.

You will notice that there is a pattern present — fewer fats in your diet equals fewer results. Most diet plans like to focus on cutting out these fats and this is what makes Keto so unique. It seems like a reasonable request to cut out fats, but when your body is left with only carbs and sugars to digest, this is actually going to be detrimental to your weight loss, your overall health and it is going to throw off your hormones. Many people come to this realization after tirelessly trying diet after diet. The Keto plan is designed to be your end-all plan, one that can work with you for the rest of your life.

Tired of Being Tired

If feeling worn out seems to be a regular pattern in your life nowadays, this is yet another reason why trying the Keto diet can benefit you. Everyone deals with their own stressors and tasks throughout the day, but the way that the body handles all of this can differ greatly. Your food is your fuel, so it makes sense that what you put into your body is super important for making it through each day. Most of us tend to feel completely drained by the end of a long day, but this doesn't have to be your standard way of feeling. When you put the right fuel into your body, it will actually create more energy than you've ever had before.

Keto can provide you with energy that lasts, not simply bursts that are fleeting. When you only receive energy in bursts, from coffee or sugar, for example, this creates the eventual feeling of a crash. This happens because the energy is only meant to be temporary and while it can get you through a moment, it isn't going to carry you throughout your whole day. The energy that Keto can give you is the energy that is more permanent. It is the kind of energy that builds up gradually, preventing you from ever feeling like you are going to crash.

In the Standard American Diet (SAD), carbs are overconsumed. In general, American's eat too many simple carbs, and unhealthy fats. Most of the time, the carb takes the center of the plate, with a side of protein, and little, if any, healthy fats. Additionally, we are junk food junkies - we eat too many processed foods that are often high in carbs and sugars, eat sugared "health" foods, like sugary/syrupy yogurt, and eat out at restaurants that dish out huge servings, loaded with terrible fats, a ton of carbohydrates. Because of this high intake of the wrong kind of carbs, these starches will actually be converted into glucose or sugar molecules.

Based on your knowledge of how the body works while it is not on a Keto diet, you can gather that your body is simply going to absorb the glucose and then use that for energy. This is where the fleeting energy problem becomes very real. In order to complete this process, your body needs insulin. As your glucose levels rise, so will your insulin. Even when your body has had enough, it continues to store the extra energy (glucose) for later. The insulin will also send your body signals to your liver that the glucose stores are now full. Assuming that your body is not insulin sensitive or insulin resistant, everything should go well.

As you age, though, your body can change in a way that will make it less able to handle its insulin levels properly. When your body realizes that it needs to catch up, it will demand itself to work even harder. Sometimes, it just isn't possible for it to do so. This is when you will find that many problems arise. You might find that you have unnecessary glucose in your bloodstream. If your body isn't burning it, then it simply collects until it gets the message to do something with it. During these periods, you will likely have your biggest surges of energy. However, these are the kind that can make you very tired after only a few hours later. These spurts of energy are ultimately not useful in the long run.

It is when your body's energy levels experience these drops that you begin feeling sluggish and start to crave more sugar and carbs. Since that is what you originally gave your body for this energy that you are receiving, it is naturally going to crave more of it. If you aren't careful, this can lead to unhealthy snacking and eating habits. You might find that you are craving quick snacks in order to get your fix and this usually means that you are going to reach for processed or artificial foods. You do not need to have insulin resistance in order to experience this. It is just the way that you are training your body by the diet that you are deciding to eat.

If you feel that you can identify with these energy highs and lows, you are not alone. So many people feel this way all the time, but they do not know how to tailor their diet in order to truly change the pattern. For most, adjusting the carbs that are consumed is not enough. This is when you will begin to feel hungry and cranky. Eating fewer carbs without replacing them is simply telling your body that you are giving it less fuel. This will begin an internal resistance that will likely leave you feeling frustrated. At the end of the day, you will probably still want to reach for those junk food favorites.

Keto is a way for you to ensure that you are properly replacing your carbs. When you follow a Keto diet based on the given percentages, you should be getting everything that you need in order to keep your energy levels steady. There should be no highs and lows, only medians that you will be able to reach. By receiving energy in this way, your body isn't going to think that this is the only energy it will receive for the day. Therefore, it will not go into a state of overworking followed by a big crash. Keto is all about balance and that is the one thing to keep in mind when you are seeking more energy.

Those who make the switch have expressed their concerns, much like concerns that you probably have. A lot of people worry that Keto just won't be enough to sustain them. They anticipate a lot of snacking and binge eating in order to correct this, but then they are pleasantly surprised when they realize that there is actually far less snacking needed throughout the day. When you are able to let go of the stigmas that surround the diet, you will find that your body will go through a natural process of adjustment. When you are changing anything, you need to make sure that you really commit to the change.

The Keto diet does drain all of your energy stores, but it replaces them with healthy fats. A lot of people assume that Keto is bad for you because it is like you are starving yourself, but that is not how it works. You are simply changing the way that your body operates and how it utilizes this energy. Your body isn't going to be angry with you for this switch like you might expect it to be. While it is an adjustment, your body is going to quickly realize that it can tap into the extra energy stores for more fuel whenever it needs to. It will learn what to do with these healthy fats that you are providing and how to make them last for long periods of time.

You will be able to say goodbye to your afternoon slumps and instead feel that you have enough energy to power through any day. There is also less of a chance that you will feel grumpy or "hangry" in between meals. Typically, when you are between meals, your body is waiting for you to give it more energy. Since your body stores this energy when you are on a Keto diet, there are reserves for it to dip into which truly allow you to experience your day without feeling like you are being distracted by hunger or cravings. Know that your transition into the Keto diet is going to vary. Depending on how carb-heavy your current diet is, it might take your body some time to retrain itself. For most people, it happens fairly quickly though. You might have to deal with a few days of an unsettled stomach before you truly begin to experience the benefits of Keto, but it should not be enough to deter you.

CHAPTER 5

Definitive Weight Loss and Increased Mental Clarity

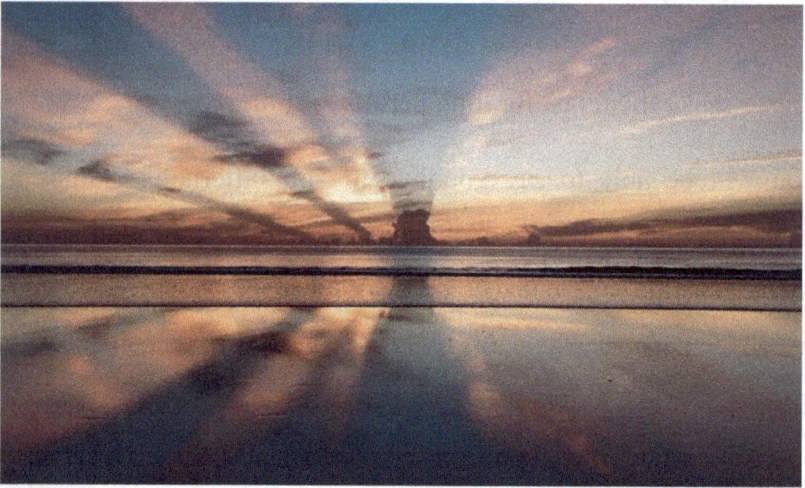

Now that you know the science behind Keto, you are likely very eager to put it to the test in your own life. With all of the benefits promised, it serves as a sustainable solution for weight management and clarity in your daily life. When your mind and body can both align, this is when you should be feeling your very best. As you begin your Keto journey, you can expect a very natural transition to take place. This is not a diet that you are going to see immediate results with, but when you start to see them, they will be long-lasting. This is not a fad diet that is going to help you shed 10lbs a week. It is a lifestyle that allows you to keep the weight off permanently. Many people who start the Keto diet have no intention of stopping and this is a healthy option if you are committed to the lifestyle.

This chapter is going to discuss what you will actually be eating while on the Keto diet. Seeing real examples of Keto-friendly menus should give you enough inspiration to create your own. When you fully understand what you should be aiming to eat, you will likely be able to think of new recipes and variations of old, familiar ones. When you are first starting out, do not have to put too much pressure on yourself to create an intricate meal plan. You can always work up to this. Having a basic and well-rounded meal plan will get you on track and it will allow you room to experiment when you feel confident enough to branch out.

Keto Ingredients

Starting out with the very basics, having knowledge about Keto-friendly ingredients is going to get you off to a good start. When you need a reminder, just think about fats and dairy. This is the basis of the diet. The following list is an example of some of the top foods that you should be reaching for while following Keto:

- Seafood (clams, muscles, oysters, squid, and octopus)

- Low-Carb Veggies (cauliflower, broccoli, and kale, leafy greens, celery, etc.)

- Cheese (especially organic, grass-fed for healthy levels of Omega 3 fatty acids)

- Avocados

- Meat and Poultry (choose grass-fed beef whenever possible, for healthy Omega 3 fatty acids)

- Eggs (choose varieties with extra Omega 3s)

- Coconut Oil (organic, extra virgin)

- Plain Greek Yogurt and Cottage Cheese (choose grass-fed for Omega 3 content)

- Olive Oil (organic, extra virgin)

- Nuts and Seeds (almonds, cashews, sunflower seeds, pecans, Macadamia nuts,

- walnuts, pistachios, pumpkin seeds, and sesame seeds)

- Berries (blueberries, raspberries, blackberries, and strawberries)

- Butter and Cream (again, preference is for grass-fed varieties for Omega 3s)

- Olives

- Unsweetened Tea and Coffee

After seeing this list of ingredients, you should be able to visualize how you can put them together in order to create nutritious meals for yourself. You can use this as a basic shopping list for your next trip to the grocery store. Shopping for your new Keto diet should not be that much different than your regular shopping trip. You have to be aware of how many carbs are in each ingredient, but otherwise, you have a lot of freedom to decide exactly what you'd like to eat for the week. For this reason, the Keto diet should never become boring or repetitive. You have so many options that you should be able to change up if necessary.

Allow yourself to explore by using some Keto-friendly ingredients in your meals that you would normally not eat on a regular basis. A handful of flax seeds in your yogurt, for example, can be a nice way to get more of your necessary nutrients without having to change the way that you would normally eat. Being crafty with these additions and substitutions will help you adjust to your new lifestyle. Eating Keto does not have to be strict and you will see just how great it will feel to be on a diet that feels like it isn't a diet. Whether you are cooking for yourself or eating outside of your home, you will be able to stick with your diet without too many issues.

Keto Food Plan

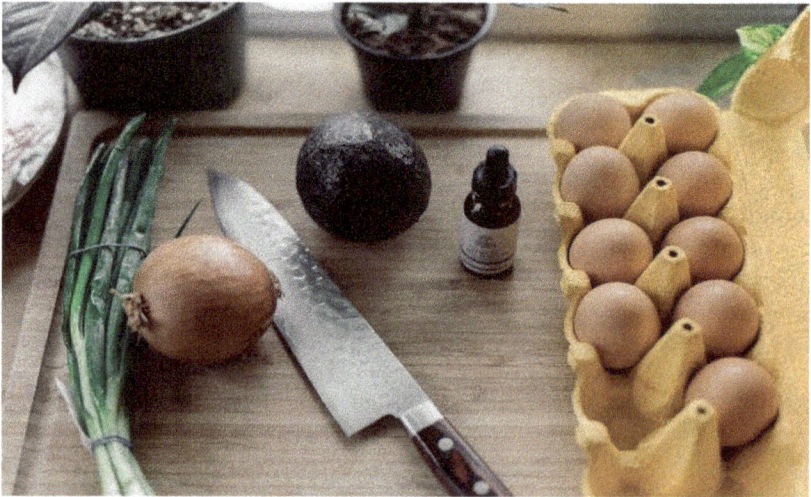

Meal planning is going to become a big part of your Keto lifestyle. When you take the time to think ahead about these things, you will feel like you are more motivated to stay on track. Deciding on what to eat when you are already really hungry is something that never goes well. When you leave it to your body to decide on this under these circumstances, this is when you are going to be most likely to give in to cravings or other unhealthy temptations that will not serve you. Meal planning is a way to keep your life organized, and while it does allow for some flexibility, it will also give you a guideline that you can continually refer to.

1st Weekly Meal Plan

	BREAKFAST	LUNCH	SNACKS	DINNER
MONDAY	Scrambled eggs with cheddar cheese, spinach, and sundried tomatoes	Cauliflower soup with bacon or tofu	Turkey and cucumber roll-ups and celery sticks with guacamole	Garlic and herb shrimp in butter sauce with zoodles (zucchini noodles)
TUESDAY	Fried eggs with sautéed greens and pumpkin seeds	Chicken salad with cucumber, avocado, tomato, onion, and almonds	Almond milk and chia seed smoothie and berries	Beef stew with mushrooms and onions
WEDNESDAY	Omelette with mushrooms, bell peppers, and broccoli	Avocado and egg salad served in lettuce cups	Mixed nuts and sliced cheese with olives and bell peppers	Cajun chicken breast with cauliflower rice and Brussels sprouts
THURSDSAY	Almond milk smoothie containing nut butter, spinach, chia seeds, and protein powder	Shrimp and avocado salad with tomatoes, feta cheese, olives, and lemon juice	Boiled eggs and flax seed crackers and cheese	Garlic butter steak with mushrooms and asparagus
FRIDAY	2 fried eggs with avocado and a side of blackberries	Grilled salmon with leafy greens and tomato	Kale chips and sliced cheese and olives	Chicken breast with cauliflower mash and a side of green beans
SATURDAY	Egg scramble with jalapeño, green onions, tomatoes, and sunflower seeds	Tuna salad with tomatoes and avocado with a side of Macadamia nuts	Celery sticks dipped in almond butter and a handful of mixed berries and nuts	Pork chops and broccoli
SUNDAY	Yogurt and granola (low-sugar) with mixed berries	Beef burger (with no bun) with guacamole, tomato, and kale salad	Sugar-free turkey jerky and an egg and vegetable muffin	Chicken stir-fry with broccoli, mushrooms, and peppers with satay sauce

Monday:

- Breakfast — Scrambled eggs with cheddar cheese, spinach, and sundried tomatoes

- Lunch — Cauliflower soup with bacon or tofu

- Dinner — Garlic and herb shrimp in butter sauce with zoodles (zucchini noodles)

- Snacks — Turkey and cucumber roll-ups and celery sticks with guacamole

Tuesday:

- Breakfast — Fried eggs with sautéed greens and pumpkin seeds

- Lunch — Chicken salad with cucumber, avocado, tomato, onion, and almonds

- Dinner — Beef stew with mushrooms and onions

- Snacks — Almond milk and chia seed smoothie and berries

Wednesday:

- Breakfast — Omelette with mushrooms, bell peppers, and broccoli

- Lunch — Avocado and egg salad served in lettuce cups

- Dinner — Cajun chicken breast with cauliflower rice and Brussels sprouts

- Snacks — Mixed nuts and sliced cheese with olives and bell peppers

Thursday:

- Breakfast — Almond milk smoothie containing nut butter, spinach, chia seeds, and protein powder

- Lunch — Shrimp and avocado salad with tomatoes, feta cheese, olives, and lemon juice

- Dinner — Garlic butter steak with mushrooms and asparagus

- Snacks — Boiled eggs and flax seed crackers and cheese

Friday:

- Breakfast — 2 fried eggs with avocado and a side of blackberries

- Lunch — Grilled salmon with leafy greens and tomato

- Dinner — Chicken breast with cauliflower mash and a side of green beans

- Snacks — Kale chips and sliced cheese and olives

Saturday:

- Breakfast — Egg scramble with jalapeño, green onions, tomatoes, and sunflower seeds

- Lunch — Tuna salad with tomatoes and avocado with a side of Macadamia nuts

- Dinner — Pork chops and broccoli

- Snacks — Celery sticks dipped in almond butter and a handful of mixed berries and nuts

Sunday:

- Breakfast — Yogurt and granola (low-sugar) with mixed berries

- Lunch — Beef burger (with no bun) with guacamole, tomato, and kale salad

- Dinner — Chicken stir-fry with broccoli, mushrooms, and peppers with satay sauce

- Snacks — Sugar-free turkey jerky and an egg and vegetable muffin

2nd Weekly Meal Plan

	BREAKFAST	LUNCH	SNACKS	DINNER
MONDAY	Scrambled eggs cooked in butter, served on top of a bed of lettuce	Spinach salad with grilled salmon	Sunflower seeds and mixed nuts	Pork chops with red cabbage slaw
TUESDAY	Coffee made with butter and coconut oil (Google "bulletproof coffee" recipes for some fun ideas) and hard-boiled eggs	Tuna salad stuffed in tomatoes	Mixed berries and Macadamia nuts	Meatballs served on zucchini noodles, topped with cream sauce
WEDNESDAY	Cheese and veggie omelette with salsa on top	Sashimi and miso soup (takeout)	Greek yogurt topped with crushed pecans and an almond milk smoothie with greens and protein powder	Roasted chicken with asparagus and sautéed mushrooms (in butter)
THURSDSAY	Almond milk smoothie with greens and protein powder	Chicken tenders served on a bed of greens with cucumbers and goat cheese	Hard-boiled eggs and sliced cheese with sliced bell peppers	Grilled shrimp topped with lemon and served with broccoli
FRIDAY	Fried eggs with bacon and a side of leafy greens	Burger in a lettuce bun, topped with avocado and served with a side salad	Walnuts with mixed berries and celery dipped in almond butter	Baked tofu with cauliflower rice, broccoli, bell peppers and a Thai peanut butter sauce
SATURDAY	Baked eggs served in avocado halves	Poached salmon and avocado rolls wrapped in seaweed	Kale chips and sugar-free jerky (turkey or beef)	Grilled beef kebabs with peppers and broccoli
SUNDAY	Scrambled eggs with veggies and salsa	Tuna salad made with mayo, served in avocado halves	Dried seaweed and cheese slices	Trout broiled with butter and sautéed bok choy

Monday:

- Breakfast — Scrambled eggs cooked in butter, served on top of a bed of lettuce

- Lunch — Spinach salad with grilled salmon

- Dinner — Pork chops with red cabbage slaw

- Snacks — Sunflower seeds and mixed nuts

Tuesday:

- Breakfast — Coffee made with butter and coconut oil (Google "bulletproof coffee recipes" for some fun ideas) and hard-boiled eggs

- Lunch — Tuna salad stuffed in tomatoes

- Dinner — Meatballs served on zucchini noodles, topped with cream sauce

- Snacks — Mixed berries and Macadamia nuts

Wednesday:

- Breakfast — Cheese and veggie omelette with salsa on top

- Lunch — Sashimi and miso soup (takeout)

- Dinner — Roasted chicken with asparagus and sautéed mushrooms (in butter)

- Snacks — Greek yogurt topped with crushed pecans and an almond milk smoothie with greens and protein powder

Thursday:

- Breakfast — Almond milk smoothie with greens and protein powder

- Lunch — Chicken tenders served on a bed of greens with cucumbers and goat cheese

- Dinner — Grilled shrimp topped with lemon and served with broccoli

- Snacks — Hard-boiled eggs and sliced cheese with sliced bell peppers

Friday:

- Breakfast — Fried eggs with bacon and a side of leafy greens

- Lunch — Burger in a lettuce bun, topped with avocado and served with a side salad

- Dinner — Baked tofu with cauliflower rice, broccoli, bell peppers, and a Thai peanut butter sauce

- Snacks — Walnuts with mixed berries and celery dipped in almond butter

Saturday:

- Breakfast — Baked eggs served in avocado halves

- Lunch — Poached salmon and avocado rolls wrapped in seaweed

- Dinner — Grilled beef kebabs with peppers and broccoli

- Snacks — Kale chips and sugar-free jerky (turkey or beef)

Sunday:

- Breakfast — Scrambled eggs with veggies and salsa

- Lunch — Tuna salad made with mayo, served in avocado halves

- Dinner — Trout broiled with butter and sautéed bok choy

- Snacks — Dried seaweed and cheese slices

When you take a look at these two sample Keto weeks, it is likely that you have identified a lot of meals that you already love and enjoy on a regular basis. This becomes a great benefit of Keto because you are likely going to be familiar with most of the food you will be eating. You don't need to completely change your tastes in order to maintain a Keto-friendly lifestyle. Most of the time, you will just need to add more of certain foods and meals that you already enjoy on a regular basis. These week-long samples should serve as some inspiration as to what you would like to be eating during a typical week.

Depending on how much time you have in your current schedule, you might find that you would rather prepare most of your meals at home. There is some variety in the menus in terms of where you will be getting your food from. Takeout is still a viable option if that is something that you already utilize in your normal lifestyle. A lot of people decide that Keto is a turning point, though. They often meal prep and plan well in advance in order to ensure that they are truly maintaining their diets. Though you can eat takeout and have meals at restaurants, you must be very careful regarding the ingredients that they are using. Modifications are almost always going to be necessary.

It is a good thing for you to be aware of these options because, sometimes, eating out is going to be your only option. Whether you are meeting with a friend for lunch or having a business meeting away from the office, there will be times when you need to eat with others. A lot of us worry that being on a diet automatically means that these fun times at restaurants must come to an end and be replaced with us sitting there without a plate of food. You don't have to give up eating in its entirety in order to eat Keto all the time! The easiest way to eat out while on Keto is to focus on your protein. Almost any restaurant you go to will have a dish that is protein-focused.

After you've found your protein of choice, determine what sides it comes with. Anything carb-heavy can usually be replaced by veggies or something that contains dairy. Make sure that you ask about these substitutions before completely ruling out the entree. If you explain to the server what you can and cannot eat, you are likely to get some recommendations as well. People go out to eat while on diets all the time and restaurants generally tend to be fairly accommodating. While you are on the Keto diet, don't be afraid to ask about modifications and substitutions. Your diet plan is important to you, so treat it that way.

If you'd rather rely on your own skills to make your Keto-friendly menu, think about how to make the process even more efficient for yourself. While some people enjoy cooking every single day, others don't have the time for it. Meal prepping can help you greatly. If you can devote a single day to your grocery shopping and meal prepping, then you can likely save a lot of time when it comes to how much cooking must be done. Try to plan your menus ahead of time, taking note of recipes that sound interesting and healthy. When you have these ideas in advance, you are likely going to be able to make faster decisions in the grocery store.

Use your meal prep time as a time to unwind. Even if cooking isn't your favorite thing to do, know that you are doing this because you are making an investment towards your health. Prepare and store all of the food that you will need for the week, dividing it into portion-controlled containers. Ideally, you should sort all of the food by meal type. This way, you will be able to simply grab a portion and go or heat it up when you need to eat something. Many Keto meal prep recipes can be eaten either hot or cold, which is helpful when you are at the office or anywhere else away from your home. You might find that the whole family will become interested in your newfound meal prep ways.

If you do want to get the entire family involved in meal planning, this serves as a great way to bond and work together to come up with the plan. Eating healthy can be difficult for many reasons, but when given options, it makes the process a lot easier. Show your family the recipes you've come up with and the ones that you have grown to love. Even if they are not on the Keto diet themselves, it is highly likely that they will find your meals just as delicious as you do. Keep a recipe book handy and add new recipes to it as you see them. When you are constantly keeping track of them, you will be more likely to remember them for later.

Remember that you can utilize a mix of both eating out and cooking for yourself when you are on Keto. The key is to take a look at your lifestyle and your current schedule in order to determine what is going to work best for you. Meal prepping can be a gradual process, so if you are only able to prep for a few days at a time, try it out this way. Nothing about eating should have to be an all or nothing process. The important thing is to pay attention to your body. If you notice that you don't feel as energized when you eat at restaurants, then you are likely not getting enough nutrition. The best way to truly give your body what it needs is by preparing the food yourself. When you can listen to your body, you will always know what you need next.

Important Note

If you are not careful, you can encounter what is known as the "Keto flu." This happens when you start the Keto diet without a proper transition into the meal plan. Its symptoms can feel similar to the standard flu and it happens as the body is getting used to digesting meals without carbs. These symptoms can vary between headaches, constipation, and nausea. While many people can successfully transition into the diet without feeling any of these things, you might go through a brief period of time when you must deal with these symptoms. One of the main ways to avoid the Keto flu is by staying hydrated. If you are dehydrated, your body is being depleted of essential minerals that it needs. When water isn't enough to hydrate you, try supplementing with sugar free electrolyte beverages.

Pre-existing conditions are also important to keep in mind. If you have conditions with your pancreas, liver, thyroid, or gallbladder, the Keto diet is not going to be suitable for you. It can also cause low blood pressure and deficiencies if you do not make sure that you keep yourself on a balanced diet. To avoid this, make sure that you are taking a multivitamin regularly. Also, it is important to note that you should avoid strenuous exercise when you get started with your diet. Allowing your body the time to transition into the Keto diet before overworking itself is essential.

CHAPTER 6

After Diet Appetite Control

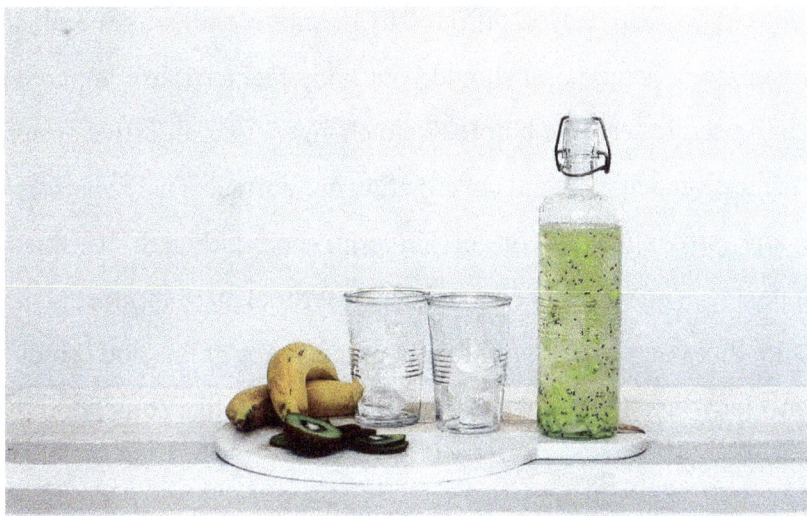

When you begin your Keto diet, an important thing to keep in mind is a method of appetite control. Any changes that are made to your normal way of eating can prompt your body to overreact and overeat. As you know, this can cause adverse effects on your body and your diet if you allow it to happen frequently. Being on any diet plan, no matter how strict or lax, requires a certain level of self-discipline. Now that you know all of the components of your Keto diet and lifestyle, you must keep them in mind at all times. When you aren't eating or snacking, your body should be in a content place. You shouldn't be craving junk food or wishing that you had more to eat. Though Keto tricks your internal systems, on a cellular level, that it is going through a period of "starvation," you should not feel this way on the outside.

Being able to recognize these red flags will ensure that you are following your Keto diet correctly. Many people wonder if it's supposed to feel bad or difficult to maintain and, in general, the answer is no. At no point should your body feel terrible compared to what it used to feel like before. Keto changes your digestive system, so some stomach pain and constipation are normal. There should not be any prolonged discomfort in your body, though. If this is happening, you might need to take a closer look at your meal plan to ensure that you are getting the right percentages of fats and proteins. Don't let yourself simply accept this bad feeling like something that is permanent.

If you find that you are getting hungry between your meals, you might need to incorporate more snacks into your diet. Snacking isn't "cheating" when you are on the Keto diet because you aren't supposed to be counting calories in a strict way. It isn't a bad thing to need snacks in order to take you from one meal to the next. It is actually a normal part of the transition from your current diet to your Keto diet. Meal prepping your snacks can be very helpful because you will always have something to reach for when you get a craving. By giving yourself only healthy and Keto-friendly snacking options, you will be less likely to stray from the path. Dividing your snacks into portion-controlled storage is also an excellent way to make sure that you are being reasonable with your cravings.

Working out might be a part of your daily lifestyle, or it might only be a part of your weekly lifestyle. No matter how often you get up and move, consider how much energy you have to burn when you do. Working out on a completely empty stomach is typically not a good idea. You will begin to feel sick or lightheaded as you get started with your workout. Try to eat something light and stay hydrated before and during your workout. After you finish up with physical activity, your body is going to need replenishment. Eating protein up to 30 minutes after a workout is going to ensure that your body has more muscle mass to build. Protein powder can also be very useful in this case, giving you a necessary boost in your smoothies before or after your workout. All you need to remember is your percentages in order to make sure that you do not overdo it with your protein intake.

Lowered Levels of Inflammation

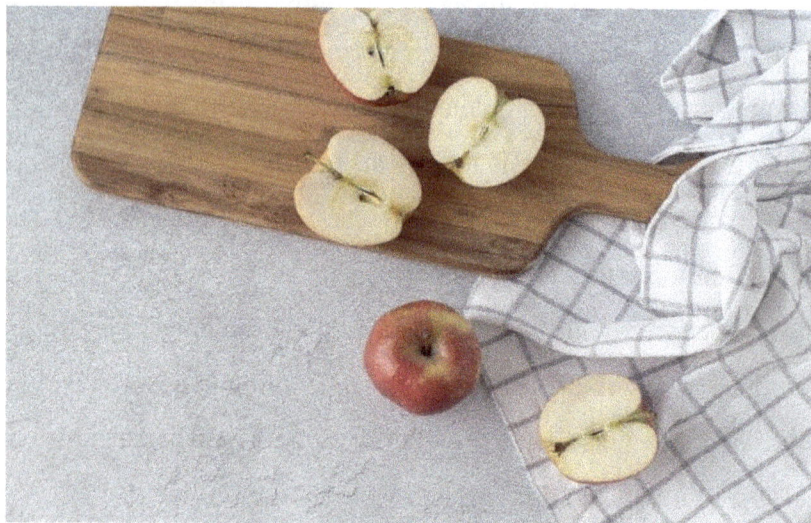

Keto is great for inflammation because it works to detoxify your body. Instead of holding on to all that sugar as it usually does, it allows your body to clean itself out. Being rid of these excess glucose stores, your body will naturally lessen the amount of inflammation that it holds onto. This is a very important benefit, especially as an aging woman because inflammation can create many problems down the road. When your joints are inflamed, many basic activities become a burden. From walking to being able to sit down in the car for longer periods of time, your body is going to be in pain if it is inflamed. Your diet has everything to do with this, as you know that the foods that are a part of the Keto plan work to combat your inflammation.

When your levels of inflammation are being properly managed by Keto, you will notice a difference when you first wake up in the morning. It is never a good idea to jump right out of bed and get moving too quickly, but that just isn't even an option when you are feeling inflamed. By getting rid of this burning and stiffness, your body will be able to adjust to being awake a lot easier. Instead of having to hit the snooze button countless times, you should be able to begin your waking up routine as soon as your alarm sounds. Get into the habit of waking up when you actually should wake up, as snoozing the alarm can create a bad start to your whole day.

Through dealing with inflammation, you have likely noticed that it gets worse when you are sitting down or standing up for long periods of time. For most of us, this means that the inflammation is at its peak while you are at work. Taking anti-inflammatory medication can be enough to dull the pain, but it usually isn't enough to keep it away for long. It is not a good feeling to be dependent on any kind of medication if you don't have to be. This is why Keto can help when it comes to an inflamed body. Instead of reaching for the medicine, you can change your eating habits to improve your inflammation. As long as you are following your Keto diet closely, it is going to begin the detoxification process right away. You should feel the impacts on your inflammation.

As you make it through your days, your body is naturally more inclined to become inflamed as you get closer to bedtime. This can prove to be very uncomfortable because you might be feeling very tired, but your inflammation is keeping you awake; maybe with restless leg syndrome, or neck and back pain. This is another point where you have likely reached for some medication in the past instead of considering what you ate for dinner. Thinking about your body as a machine that needs the right oils to operate can help you stay on track with your Keto diet. While there are always going to be temptations waiting around every corner, when you think about just how good Keto is going to make you feel, this should make it worthwhile to stick to the plan.

Inflammation is a natural part of aging. There isn't much that you can do to avoid it altogether, but preventative measures will help you in the long run. You can think of the Keto diet as a preventative approach. While it is a great diet plan, it also serves as a way to maintain your physical health by keeping you protected from these various ailments. You deserve to be on a diet that allows you to feel great *and* look great. Keto isn't simply about vanity. It allows you to get your health back on track, even if you have been unhealthy for the last several years. A common misconception is that there comes a point when it is too late to make a healthy change — it is never too late.

When you begin to live your life without your body resting in a state of inflammation, you will realize how much easier your day-to-day activities become. Starting with sleeping, you will be able to have a more restful night of sleep when your body isn't inflamed. This means that you will also be able to wake up earlier and have a more productive start to your day. Many things that you are able to accomplish happen when your body gets enough rest. If you are overworking yourself and then not making up for it with the food that you eat, you are just going to feel fatigued and down all the time.

With less inflammation also comes more potential to workout. While you don't need a bodybuilder routine, you know that getting enough physical activity into each week is an important part for any woman over 50. Staying moving will keep your body working correctly; our bodies are designed to be in motion, and not sedentary. The Keto diet will also boost your metabolism and increase your energy levels. What you will realize is that everything in your body is connected, even if it doesn't always seem this way. Less inflammation means fewer burdens, in general. Make note of how you feel before and after your Keto diet begins. The results will likely amaze you. The best part is, there are no gimmicks in sight. Keto just works with your body.

Clean Food for a Clean Mindset

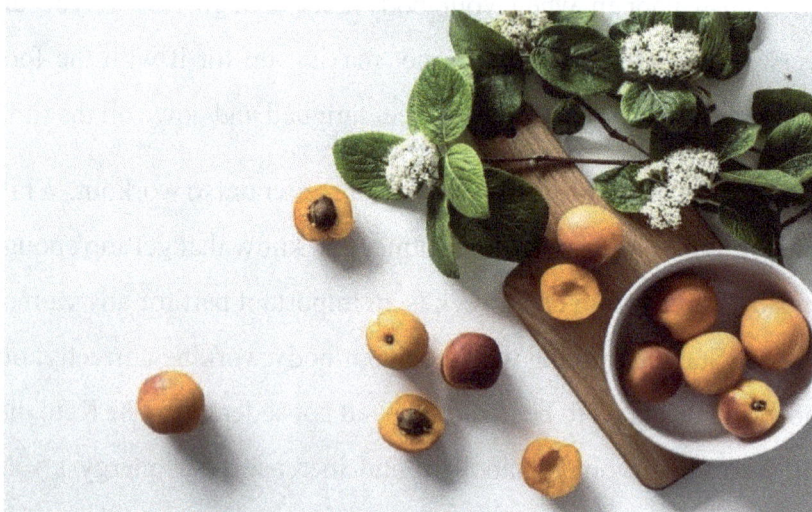

You are likely familiar with the term "clean eating," but how does that fit into your new Keto lifestyle? The principle behind eating clean is that you should aim to eat natural, whole foods whenever possible. Instead of selecting pre-packaged ingredients that contain preservatives or additives, and extra fats, sugars and salt, eating clean promotes you to only use fresh ingredients. While this can be time-consuming and difficult for those who are not used to it, eating clean will prove to be worthwhile. When your body is used to digesting real and organic food, there is less room for it to absorb any unhealthy sugars or fats. When you eat clean, you digest clean. This also allows you to have a clearer mindset.

If you aren't eating clean already, then you are likely settling yourself short when it comes to getting enough nutrients. Only natural foods have the right amount of nutrients to properly fuel your body. Even if you are eating a canned and preserved vegetable, you aren't going to be getting nearly as many nutrients as you would from eating the fresh version. It is through small changes like these that will allow you to make healthier and cleaner choices. While you don't have to opt for the organic-only grocery store, you can start by working on these smaller details.

Thinking about the foods that you are encouraged to eat while on the Keto diet, it makes sense that you are going to take a cleaner approach. In order to prepare your proteins and vegetables, it takes a simple strategy. With the occasional addition of butter or dairy, these are the ingredients that you will use to flavor the rest of the food. When you buy meat, make sure that it is always fresh. If you do have to freeze it for later, be sure to correctly label it in your freezer so it will not go bad before you get the chance to use it. Any vegetables that you will be eating on the Keto diet can be purchased fresh. It doesn't really make sense to opt for the canned versions because the fresh ones are going to taste better while providing a more nourishing benefit. If you can't get fresh vegetables, frozen veggies are a much better option than canned.

Another benefit that you can gain from eating clean comes from the knowledge that you will have access to. Being aware of what exactly is in the food that you are eating becomes an essential part of your Keto diet. When you eat clean, you will know how much protein, fat, and carbs you will be getting from eating certain foods. Not only do you need to know this information to stay on track with your Keto diet, but it also becomes helpful for you to know in general. Having an awareness of what you are eating and what it is doing to your body is very important.

Eating clean also means eating locally as much as possible. When you can utilize the ingredients in your local area, you are supporting these smaller farms as well as reducing your carbon footprint. It takes a lot of resources in order to mass-produce food which is why it makes more sense to utilize the local resources that are readily available. The planet does not have an endless supply of food, so when we can be smarter with the way that we eat, it is going to make a difference for the future. Do your best to seek out farmer's markets whenever possible. There are likely a few in your local area for you to explore. You might even discover some foods that you have never tried before because they are not typically available in regular grocery stores.

As mentioned, eating clean can also benefit your mindset. This becomes possible because of the way that eating good food can impact how you are feeling mentally. When you are eating wholesome ingredients, your body is going to respond well to this. Not only will you feel better physically, but your mental health will also see improvement. You will be able to think clearer and in a more positive way. It is almost as though your mind also goes through the same detoxification process as your body. With a clearer mind, you will see yourself doing better with various social interactions and work responsibilities. Your brain will be as sharp as it can as you navigate through all of the mental tasks that you must face each day.

If you think about it, clean eating is a savorier experience. If you were to reach for your favorite fast food burger, you would likely eat it pretty quickly. Now, imagine eating a salad with all of your favorite ingredients on it. Which one would take you longer to eat? The salad would, likely due to the fact that you have to slow down to eat it. Fast food isn't always the better option. We should not be focused on eating fast because this is actually detrimental to our physical health. When we are able to slow down the eating process and truly savor our food, we are also able to digest it better. When your body is working at a slower rate, it will know exactly how it needs to process what you are eating. Instead of eating just to simply fill yourself up, think about what your body needs. Consider what kind of fuel you can give yourself in order to be the best version of yourself possible. You'll be glad that you slowed down.

CHAPTER 7

Food for Stable Blood Sugar Levels

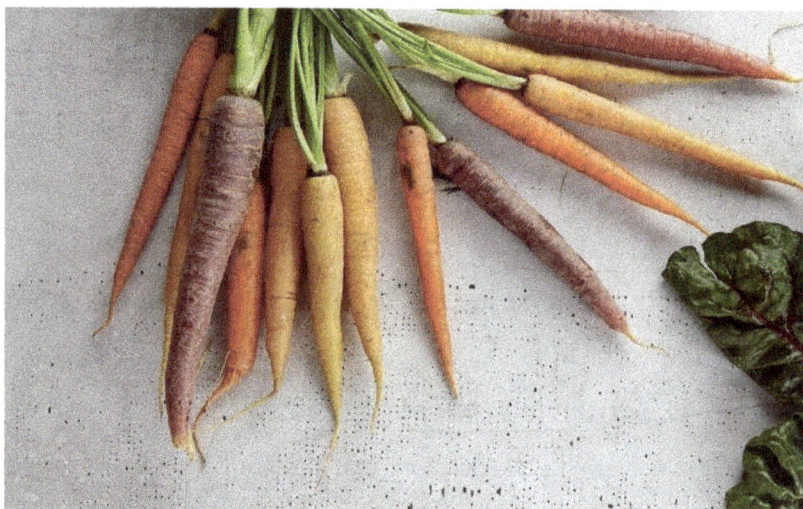

When you eat, you are likely only thinking about one thing — satisfying your hunger. While this is a big part of what eating is, it is not the only factor. The older we get, the less stable our blood sugars become. This happens naturally, and sometimes, it is to no fault of your own. The aging process isn't very forgiving unless you make an effort to manage it. If you simply allow your body to age and continue to feed it foods that do not properly nourish it, then you aren't going to be feeling the best you can feel. Eating should be a way for you to stabilize your energy levels, by keeping blood sugars in balance. It should fill you up while also replenishing your needs.

If you eat junk food, you get one of these aspects. Being full is not the same thing as being healthy, though.

Consider the last meal that you ate and think about how full you got from it. Did you feel so full that you wished you hadn't eaten as much? How satisfying was the meal overall? Did you get hungry again soon after eating? These questions are all helpful tools in gauging how healthy you are with your meal choices. Even if your meals contain healthy ingredients, this does not automatically mean that you are eating in the healthiest way possible. The Keto diet helps you to reframe the way that you eat. It allows you to have large, satisfying portions while promoting clean eating simultaneously. This diet should keep you feeling healthy at all times.

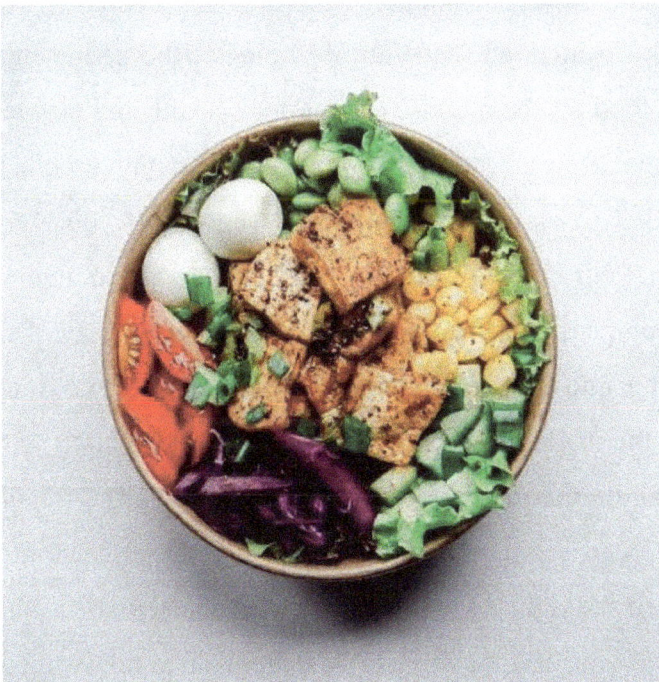

You are no stranger to the connection between carbs and blood glucose by now. When you partake in the Keto diet, you should also know how it works to eliminate this excess sugar in order to keep your body healthier. What you must keep in mind is that Keto is designed to manage your blood sugar levels, not eliminate them. We still need this glucose in order to survive. When you eat Keto-friendly foods, you are not aiming to get rid of it all in its entirety. Instead, you are aiming for a more balanced level in your body. When you have too much or too little of anything that your body makes naturally, this is going to cause you to have health problems. This is why sticking to the percentages of the Keto diet is so important. They will keep you healthy and functional, ensuring that you do not deplete your body of anything in the process.

Again, keep in mind that you are going to be eating this Keto-friendly food for the purpose of long-term health and wellness. You do not actually want to deprive yourself of anything while you are on the diet or else it will not work properly. If you are lacking anything, your body is going to send out signals that might force it to overcompensate. When it has to focus on this instead of focusing on getting into a state of ketosis, then your body is going to be missing the mark when it comes to eating Keto. This is why many people agree that eating Keto takes preparation. By reading this guide, you are taking the steps necessary that you need in order to get started the right way. When you are educated about the diet to the best of your ability, you will be better able to follow it correctly.

If you are too restrictive while on the Keto diet, this can cause your body to become insulin sensitive. This happens when the body stops producing as much glucose, therefore producing less insulin. Remember, none of the different versions of the Keto diet ask you to cut out carbs completely. While you are going to be eating a fraction of the amount that you once ate, you are still going to be getting some in your system in order to prevent these health issues. A lot of people who are unsure about the Keto diet tend to believe that the body is going to run into these problems while attempting to eat fewer carbs. Balance is everything when it comes to dieting and as long as you are following the recommended carb consumption, then you should be just fine.

On the other end of the diet, if you do not follow it closely enough, then your body isn't going to start producing and storing less glucose. This usually happens when people try to follow the diet, but do not have the willpower to keep going. This can actually be more damaging to your body than not starting Keto at all. If you are going to be doing things halfway, then you should hold off until you feel that you are ready to truly commit to the diet. You cannot expect to follow some of the rules yet get the same great results and benefits. Being realistic with your approach is going to save you from the discouragement and the hassle of not seeing the results that you are expecting.

If you ever feel that you are losing sight of your diet and what you should be eating, take a moment to regroup. Think about the benefits of the Keto diet and use them as motivation in order to keep eating properly. Cravings are natural and they will come during various points of your week. Knowing how to acknowledge them while not giving in to them will allow you to stay focused. When your blood sugar levels are changing, your body might send signals to your brain saying that it needs sugar. Know that this is just a cry for help, but that your body is going to adjust on its own in order to start burning energy from fats instead. Keep yourself calm by remembering why you are on the Keto diet in the first place and filling up on foods that are packed with healthy fats and protein instead.

Clean Food for Powerful Living

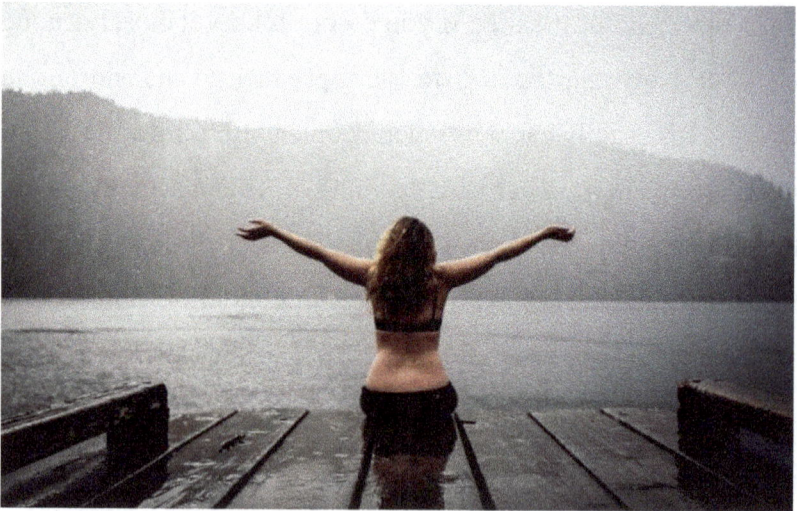

The Keto diet can definitely be thought of as a method for detoxification. In order to detox, this does not mean that you need to be empty and starving. What it means is that you are giving your body the chance to eat the purest ingredients that are free of artificial ingredients. This goes back to what we discussed earlier, with clean living, but worth a little deeper insight.

When you are choosing foods that are packaged and processed - think natural — if you can't pronounce it, then you likely don't need to be consuming it. While a lot of additives are in place to preserve the quality of the food that we eat, they are not necessarily supposed to be consumed on a regular basis. While there isn't immediate danger behind occasionally eating processed foods, your body is going to get used to them. When this happens, it makes it harder for you to switch to a clean method of eating.

Without the presence of additives, your body can take everything that you eat and turn it into something useful. Instead of having to sort through what is nourishment and what is filler, and what needs to be filtered or cleaned by your liver, your body is going to be able to go straight into the process of converting fats into energy. It will have a purpose that is clear and guided. The Keto diet aims to help provide your body with this necessary clarity. Because it does not include any ingredients that are unnecessary for your consumption, you can rest assured knowing that everything you eat is going to have its own purpose and intended use. Your body will automatically know what to do when you give it these natural ingredients to work with.

Research suggests that everyone can benefit from a detox in their diet. Even if it isn't going to be a permanent change, devoting a week or two via clean eating can do a lot in order to reset your system. The great thing about the Keto diet is that it gives you a chance to feel the benefits of a detox without having to commit to many restrictions. Most people think about going on juice cleanses when they hear the word detox, but this isn't the only way to make it happen. Just like anything else, there are levels to the process. You can detox your body while still eating just as much, if not more, food that you are used to eating.

The cravings that you will experience while you are on the Keto diet are going to challenge you. There is no way to avoid them completely, but you can be sure to build up your tolerance toward them the more you work at it. Believe it or not, the cravings do subside over time. When your body is able to detox all of the sugar from your system, it will forget what it feels like to crave it. While you will have to deal with a short period of cravings, your body is eventually going to begin craving other things. You might notice a shift in craving sugar to craving protein instead. Many people never end up trying the Keto diet because they believe that their bodies are simply going to crave sugar the whole time. If you can work your way through these initial cravings, you will find that it is actually a lot easier than you think to keep these cravings managed.

It is simply a matter of changing bad habits to good habits and shifting your mindset from the negative to the positive. This is a natural transition whenever we are changing our lifestyle, and in some ways, we're hard-wired to resist change. So, let's take a look at some ways to tackle this very common issue.

CHAPTER 8

Changing Your Habits and Your Mindset to Change Your Body

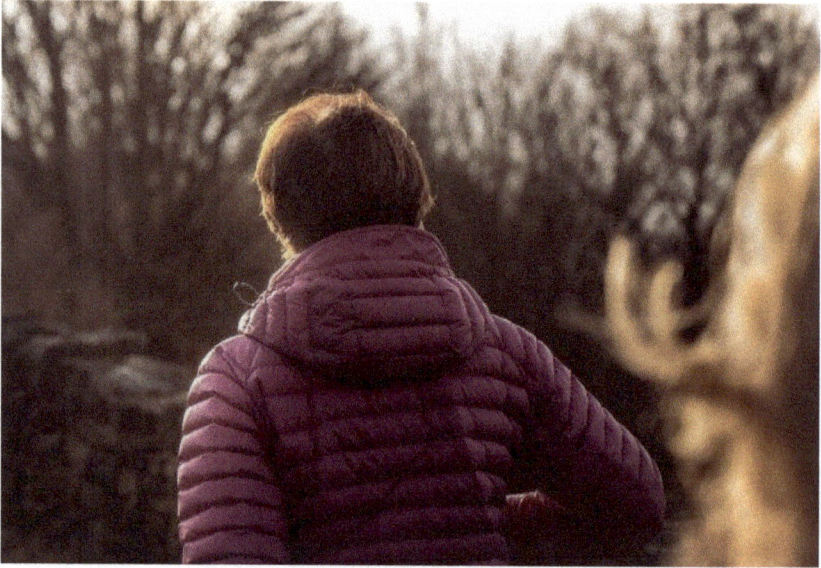

Being on a diet means following guidelines. When you already have guidelines in place, it becomes a process to switch between your current one and your new one. Try not to think about your Keto diet as a lifestyle change that is going to limit you. If you are able to see it as something that is a healthy and positive change, you are going to have a better mindset while beginning the diet. By having a clear understanding of what you should be eating and how you should be feeling, you can compare the way that you feel to the way that the diet is supposed to make you feel. This allows you to stay in control of your diet without feeling that you have to completely surrender all of your decision-making.

We all have our own bad habits, and a lot of us have bad eating habits. In today's society, it becomes easy to fall into these habits because of the promise of convenience. If you had the choice to get takeout or make a meal for yourself in a hurry, you would likely opt for takeout because you have been trained to believe that it is faster and easier. While it might be faster, you are likely compromising the quality of the food that you are eating because it appears more convenient. Most of the time, it doesn't take that much additional effort to cook for yourself. With the way that society pushes fast food and various food delivery services, it is no wonder that you would be more comfortable with allowing someone else to make your food.

While some of these services can be incredibly convenient, you are settling yourself short because you do not know exactly what you are eating. You do not know where the ingredients are from and how they were prepared. These things matter to your overall health, especially as aging becomes a factor. More than ever, you need to be paying attention to the source of your food. When you let these decisions go out of your control, you are allowing others to decide what is best for your body. Even when you begin to feel sluggish and less functional, the body becomes easily addicted to junk food so it will trick you into thinking that you need to keep eating this way.

This chapter puts focus on the things that you are already doing and how you can change them for your own health. It is hard to change your habits, but it is not impossible. As long as you have the motivation and the drive to keep moving forward, then you should be able to see real results. It often takes years to form a bad habit, so don't be discouraged if you don't notice a difference immediately. This part does take some time, but each time that you put effort into it, you are going to be working toward your main goal of becoming healthier. Tell yourself that you are doing this for your own benefit. Any time that things feel too difficult, try to get yourself back on track by remembering how great you feel when you are eating natural food that optimizes your health.

How to Make Changes: Step by Step

It becomes easier said than done when you are asked to change your eating habits. Even if you know exactly what your end result should look like, it can often be difficult to get from point A to point B. The trick is to break this part down into daily steps. You can't just expect yourself to adjust to these changes right away. The body and the mind both need time to process the changes in order to accept them as what is new and preferred. If you can commit to working on these habits each day, then you have already completed step one. Being committed to the cause is going to allow you to see real results. If you are only halfway interested in succeeding, you can imagine your results to look the same.

Start with Breakfast

You can start one meal at a time when you are planning on working on your eating habits. Think about how you start your day. Do you eat breakfast, or do you opt to wait until lunch comes around? If you choose not to eat breakfast, yet you are consuming a lot of snacks until lunch, this can become a detrimental habit. Even if you do eat breakfast, if you are loading up on sugars and carbs, this can also prove to have some negative results. Eating a balanced breakfast is how you are going to have a balanced day ahead. Your breakfast should be your fuel from the time you walk out the door until you are able to sit down and have your lunch. As you know, many will agree that breakfast is the most important meal of the day.

Even if you don't feel extremely hungry in the morning, try to eat something that will provide you with nutrition. A heavy breakfast isn't necessary but getting some protein in your body before you start your day will result in a noticeable difference. Keto breakfasts are great because they can vary in size. A lot of people feel minimal hunger when they first wake up and that is okay. Try to at least get into the habit of consuming a smoothie so that you have something in your stomach. After doing this for a week straight, you should notice that your energy levels are higher. You will also have more focus at the beginning of your day.

Stay Hydrated

As you make your way through each day, keep track of how much water you are drinking. No matter what diet you are on, drinking water is always going to be the best beverage option. Keto encourages you to drink as much water as possible. When you are hydrated, all of your bodily systems work a lot better. Water also gives you energy and fills you up when you start to have cravings. Although water cannot truly make you feel full, it can sustain you and make you feel great in between meals. If you are doing anything that is physically taxing, it is especially important to stay hydrated. As the body ages, it starts to need more hydration at a quicker pace. If you start feeling symptoms of the "keto flu," make sure you hydrate with electrolytes (sugar-free).

Avoid Sugary Drinks

If you choose a drink other than water, you need to pay attention to how much sugar it contains. Even natural fruit juices can be high in natural sugars. One of the main points of Keto is to avoid sugar, so you will have to be careful with your selection. This is why choosing water can be a simple fix because you never have to worry about how much sugar you are consuming. For a lot of people, getting rid of sodas and juices that are filled with high fructose corn syrup can be hard. Anything that you are used to becomes hard to give up. You can try flavoring your water naturally if you need some motivation to drink it. Infuse your water with fruits for a nice added flavor.

Healthy Lunches

Think about what you can change during lunchtime. Something that matters a great deal, but people often fail to think about is the speed at which they consume their lunches. Many people will eat lunch at work or away from home and this usually happens on a timed break. If you are also in this situation, keep in mind that you shouldn't have to rush to eat your lunch. This is when you might accidentally overeat or eat too much of the wrong thing in an attempt to nourish your body. Meal planning can come in handy for lunchtime especially because you will already have a balanced meal without having to worry about it. If you don't already, consider bringing a pre-packed lunch to work.

Keto Outside the Home

You are bound to have at least a few meals outside of your home and this is definitely possible with the Keto diet, as you know. The same exact rules are going to apply, so it is up to you to request changes when necessary. If something comes with a side of carbs, ask if you can make substitutions. In many cases, you can mention that you are on the Keto diet and people will likely understand what it is that you can and cannot eat. However, when you are trying to follow any diet plan, it is your responsibility to correctly inform others who are going to be preparing your food. By explaining that you can only eat fats and dairy, there should be minimal confusion about how you need to avoid carbs.

Don't be afraid to speak up when you are eating outside of your home. This is the number one way that diets get ruined because it seems like an inconvenience to make changes. If you are truly going to commit to Keto, you need to make sure that you are monitoring your own diet. No one else is going to do this for you, which makes it even more of a victory when you can keep it up without breaking the guidelines. While Keto isn't a strict diet, you do need to be firm with yourself when you go out to eat. Sometimes, being in the presence of friends or loved ones can be tempting. If they are all eating something that you wish you could be eating, it becomes easier for you to convince yourself that you can have it too. Remember, one slip-up can mean that your body isn't going to enter ketosis. This means that the Keto diet will no longer be working the way it should.

This isn't to say that eating with others is a bad thing. Yes, you are going to have to deal with temptations, but you can still enjoy a group eating experience while still sticking to your Keto diet. When you explain to your loved ones what the diet consists of and why, they are likely going to be more sensitive to the things that you are trying to avoid. When you aren't being offered carbs and sugars, you have a higher chance of being able to forget about them and will not end up craving them as frequently. Eating around others can boost your morale because it shows you the most enjoyable parts of the experience. When you can focus on the social aspect of eating, you will end up enjoying it a lot more than if you were to focus on what you *can't* have.

Time Meals Strategically

Understand that you need time to digest your dinner. A meal that is typically eaten at home, you need to make sure that you aren't eating too close to bedtime. Since Keto does consist of a lot of meat-eating, this can feel very heavy if you are eating too late at night. When you pick a dinner time, try to stick with it. This will get your body used to digesting at a certain speed and it will get you into a regular routine. Getting into these routines is great on the Keto diet because they will keep you regulated. Try to focus on getting your nutrition in and then partaking in gentle activities. You should never eat right before you are about to lie in bed. This can upset your stomach and tell your body that it is done digesting when it actually isn't. As a result, you will likely experience insomnia or restlessness.

Keto Snacking

Change the way that you view snacking. If you have any negative connotations regarding eating snacks, you should know that this isn't necessary when you are on the Keto diet. Not only are there many Keto-friendly snacks that you can prepare for yourself, but snacking is also a very valid way to get you from meal to meal. As your body is transitioning the way that it utilizes energy, you might end up eating more snacks than you've ever eaten. This is okay! As long as you are keeping nourishing options available, then you should not be in danger of breaking your diet. A snack isn't going to fill you up like a meal will, but it should be able to hold you over until you are able to fully nourish yourself. If you are going to be out of your house for a while, it is advised that you bring a snack or two along. This will prevent you from buying food that is unhealthy for you.

Meal Prepping

Keep a recipe book in your kitchen. You can gather your favorite Keto-friendly meal ideas in one place. This way, if you ever have to prepare a meal on the spot or if you need meal prep ideas, you won't have to search for very long. You can always keep your eyes open for different recipes that you would like to try. Categorize your recipe book by the ones that you have tried and love to the ones that you would like to try in the future. If you wanted to, you could also categorize them by meal type or cuisine type. You can have a lot of creative freedom when it comes to the way that you do this, so experiment all you want! When you make it a habit to become more comfortable in the kitchen, you are going to notice this in the quality of the meals that you create.

Building New Habits - One Meal at a Time

All of these ideas are fairly simple, but they will encourage you to make important changes. Much like you had to make some changes to begin the Keto diet, you can continue to make changes in your daily life to improve your diet. Getting into a healthier mindset doesn't always happen right away, but the more that you practice, the easier it will become. You will be able to show yourself that you can manage your diet while you are away from home and you will be able to control your cravings when they hit. As long as you can keep a solid foundation, you will always be able to return to it when you need to. Keep yourself motivated by reminding yourself how you are getting healthy both inside and out.

CHAPTER 9

Reaching Your Goal

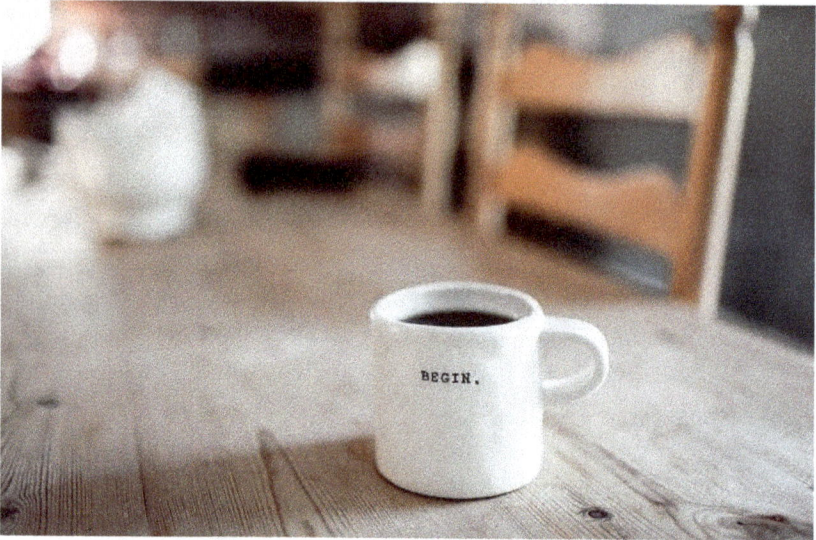

The saying remains true — you will realize that what you put into your body is going to dictate how you feel. While on the Keto diet, you are building up energy stores for your body to utilize. This means that you should be feeling a necessary boost in your energy levels and the ability to get through each moment of each day without struggling. You can say goodbye to the sluggish feeling that often accompanies other diet plans. When you are on Keto, you should only be experiencing the benefits of additional energy and unlimited potential. Your diet isn't going to always feel like a diet. After some time, you will realize that you actually enjoy eating a

Keto menu very much. Because your body is going to be switching the way it metabolizes, it will also be switching what it craves. Don't be surprised if you end up craving fats and proteins as you progress on the Keto diet — this is what your body will eventually want.

Tracking Progress

Using a compare and contrast method is always great for tracking progress. Remember how you felt prior to starting the Keto diet. If you haven't started already, you can use this time to document your current state of being. Make sure to record your mindset and the cravings that you have. You can also mark down your current weight and BMI. When you have these figures to compare your progress to, you will be able to use this as a motivating tool. Remember to allow yourself the feeling of pride as you make it through each day of being on the Keto diet. Make a commitment to yourself and to the diet. This is going to present its own set of challenges to face, but they are not going to be so difficult that you lose your way. Believe in your ability to see this through.

You Are What You Eat

Think about how you used to feel while eating your sugary and carb-loaded cravings. Your immediate response is likely going to suggest that you felt great but think about the bigger picture. Did you gain more energy from eating these things? Did you experience a crash after you ate them? Instant gratification might feel great at first, but you will likely have to deal with the consequences after the fact. Eating junk food only serves your immediate cravings. It also gets your body used to craving these things by reinforcing the behavior. Junk food holds no nutritional value and it won't make you burn calories or use the sugar as a valid energy supply. When you think about it, this junk food truly doesn't have a place in your life.

Know that you can obtain happiness in other ways that don't involve eating food. While eating does tend to be a social delight, it isn't the only thing that can make you happy when it comes to food. Choose to feel happy when you can know for certain that you are treating your body properly. You should be able to feel the joy that comes from the fact that you are giving your body fuel that it can actually utilize. While eating your Keto-friendly food might not give you the same immediate rush that eating your favorite junk food does, it will benefit you much more in the long run. You will be able to notice its benefits long after you digest the food and that is what is important. A simple change in perspective is what you need to realize that your happiness isn't directly tied to the cravings that you satisfy. Your happiness needs to stem from a deeper place.

Eating tends to be an act of comfort when you are feeling down or worried. This is a cultural norm that many people experience. While being on the Keto diet, you will learn how to manage your emotions in a way that is not directly tied to the food you are eating. Instead of giving in to your cravings when you are having a hard day, the Keto diet teaches you to nourish yourself instead. When you are properly nourished, you will be able to boost your energy levels and maintain your endorphins. As you know, this will be enough to give you some extra happiness when you need it. It is a more permanent solution to your problems that tend to linger. When you can think about things from this perspective, it will be easier to remember why you are on the Keto diet at all.

No diet should make you feel so miserable that you can't even enjoy its benefits. Keto is definitely not a diet that should make you feel like you have no options. While on Keto, you should actually have the exact opposite experience. Because what you have to get rid of is so minimal, you should be equipped with many different meals that you can enjoy on a guilt-free level. Diets that torment you emotionally are not good for you, no matter how healthy you are eating. Having a healthy mind is just as important as having a healthy body. When your mindset begins to deteriorate, this will lessen your overall happiness levels. You are allowed to be happy while being on a diet! If you start to feel down, then something isn't right.

Through your example, other people will begin to see that Keto isn't as strict or difficult as they once thought. Being able to provide others with a real perspective can do a lot to keep the diet realistic. You can serve as an inspiration to your friends and loved ones with the way that you are able to stick with your diet and remain happy and fulfilled. You may have likely tried to fake this feeling while being on diets in the past, but Keto does not involve any pretending. It is important to listen to exactly how you are feeling and identify what is making you feel this way. If you begin to experience anything negative, you are encouraged to alter your diet until you begin to feel better. There should be no suffering while on the Keto diet!

Your Life Will Improve

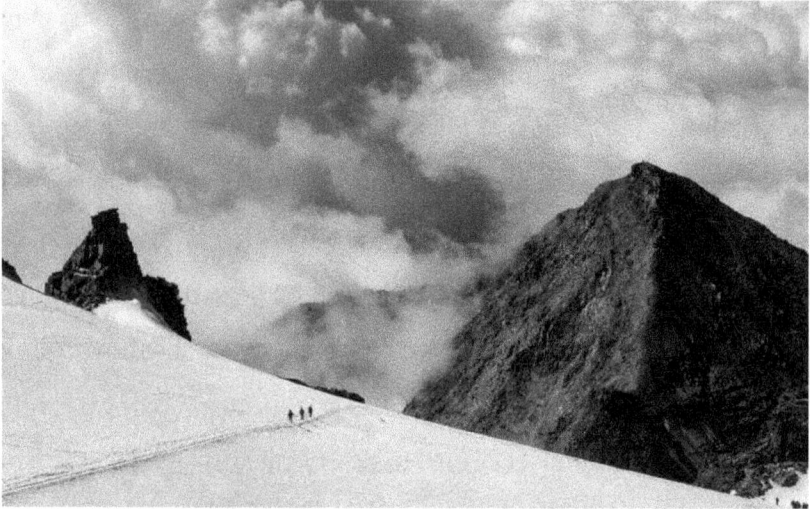

There comes a point while being on the Keto diet that you make a shift from trying to succeeding. This will happen at various points for people, but when it happens to you, embrace it. Instead of focusing on the fact that you are following a diet, you can begin to shift your focus to the benefits that you are receiving. You need to make sure that you are enjoying your life! There are so many things in life that try to get you down, so when you find something that actually brings you up, you should focus your attention on these things. One of the very first things that the Keto diet will provide you with is energy. As you have read, this is one of the benefits that you should experience fairly quickly. Use your energy to the best of your ability. Try to divide your time wisely, keeping in mind that the diet has allowed you some additional fuel to use throughout your day.

Even if you feel that your energy levels are currently on the rise, try to still practice healthy habits like going to bed earlier and waking up earlier. This is going to further regulate your bodily systems. What you need to remember is that the Keto diet is going to give you momentum. It is up to you to keep up with it. If you do nothing with it, then it is almost like these benefits are being wasted. When you can remain aware of them, you should be able to take full advantage of them. Try to practice as many healthy habits as you can when you first start noticing these new changes. This can be a very exciting and uplifting time for you!

Your Body Will Change

One of the next benefits that you will begin enjoying is the way that your appearance will change. Your skin should have a healthy glow to it, appearing youthful. As the aging process takes place, feeling ashamed of your skin can become a prominent issue that impacts your self-esteem greatly. Don't feel upset because your body is doing what it is supposed to be doing naturally. Aging is a process that no one is exempt from, but the Keto diet can help you do it more gracefully. When you notice that your skin is improving, you can make a commitment to taking better care of it. Make sure that you go to bed each night with a clean face, wear sunscreen daily, and moisturize on a regular basis. It doesn't take much to ensure that you have a solid skincare routine, so do your best to treat your skin as best as you can.

Of all the changes that Keto brings, the weight loss is probably the most anticipated. When you first begin to lose weight, you are going to feel a wave of excitement wash over you. It will become a personal challenge to keep losing weight and to keep maintaining your health. Because you are going to be burning actual fat, this weight loss isn't just a temporary experience. As long as you keep up with the Keto diet, you should be able to confidently keep the weight off with ease. Many other diets will show you quick weight loss results, but that only happens because you are losing water weight, or worse - muscle. This kind of weight tends to be a lot easier to put back on, therefore creating some discouraging results.

Whether you started the Keto diet to lose weight or to just get healthier, your body is going to begin slimming down. If you want to build muscle in the process, you need to time your workouts properly and ensure that you are getting enough physical activity each week. Knowing what forms of exercise, you enjoy will allow you to have a great workout experience. If you aren't a bodybuilder, you shouldn't have to put yourself through a bodybuilder workout routine. It just wouldn't make sense. You need to make sure that your workout plan is appropriate for your current lifestyle and experience level. You can always adjust it in the future to give yourself more of a challenge if you wish.

An often overlooked benefit to starting Keto is that you are actually going to gain a lot of experience in the kitchen. Since your meals will have to be modified, it becomes a lot easier to prepare them all yourself. While you will occasionally have meals that are prepared for you, you'll find that cooking can become a fun process. You will be learning about new food combinations and new ways to flavor the same food that you know and love. Even if you have minimal cooking experience, you should be able to create a simple Keto menu for yourself that doesn't take too much time to complete. If you work on this enough, you will start feeling more confident in the kitchen, possibly even preparing the same meals for other members of the household.

Your diet doesn't make you who you are. This is why it is possible to still enjoy every part of your life while being on Keto. The way that you eat makes up a big portion of your life, it isn't your entire life. Think about all of the other great qualities that you have that are unrelated to the Keto diet. This will make you appreciate yourself more and see that Keto is simply going to be providing you with additional benefits. You already have plenty of amazing qualities to celebrate, even without this diet. Keeping these two things separate will limit any feelings of guilt or failure when you are struggling to stay on your diet. Know that there is no diet out there that is worth destroying your self-worth over.

Having a healthy relationship with dieting is going to allow you to become your most successful version of yourself. If you start the Keto diet and end up loathing it, this isn't going to give you the best results. Your diet should be a positive addition to your life, not a burden that distresses you. Diet culture tends to teach you that you must battle with your diet in order to make it work for you. Keto is so different because there should never be this kind of a struggle. Since you are constantly listening to your body and your mind, you should only be feeling positive things.

If you are ever unsure if the Keto diet is working for you, consider all of the above factors that were discussed. Are you experiencing these benefits while still being able to enjoy your life in the way that you want to? Any time you feel limited, it is because you are unnecessarily putting these limits on yourself. Try to lighten up if you begin to feel this way. You will be able to teach yourself that it is possible to be on the Keto diet without upholding this strict sense of being. Remind yourself that you are a whole person, diet or no diet. Keto should not define you, but instead, enhance all of your great qualities. When you can realize this, you will be able to see that you are thriving. It is a fantastic feeling to know that your goals are being met and you are feeling great while doing so.

Your efforts should not only inspire those around you, but they should also serve as a way to inspire yourself. Acknowledge your progress and recognize the challenges that you had to face while arriving there. Being on a diet isn't the easiest experience at first, but you will find that you can adapt to Keto seamlessly. You will wonder what you even used to eat before. This is why Keto tends to be a permanent solution. Even those who agree to try it for a few months end up sticking with it for much longer. You should keep it up unless it no longer feels good. If you are getting all of your benefits plus the satisfaction of being full of eating clean foods, then you are likely going to continue feeling great while on Keto.

CHAPTER 10

Charged with Optimism

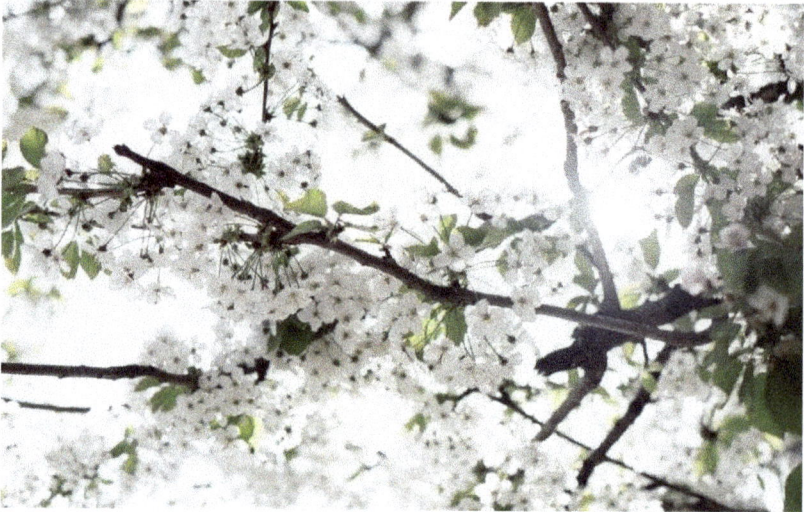

Optimism is a feeling that you will get used to while eating a Keto diet. It is a way of being that showers you with positivity in every aspect of your life. While you are going to always face challenges and setbacks in your life, having an optimistic outlook is going to help guide you through anything that you encounter. Certain things can feel discouraging the older that you get because it becomes harder to correct them. Taking care of your body and losing weight can be a couple of those things. If you no longer have hope that you can accomplish certain things, then it is not going to be easy to stay optimistic. This is how being on the Keto diet can help you. Everything that it does for your body aligns with an optimistic outlook. Because you will be taking care of your mind and body, this leaves little room for pessimism.

Before you even begin your diet, it is a wise idea to reevaluate your life. Think about what you do to cope with things when they get difficult. You might find that your coping abilities are not up to par when you realize that they revolve around eating poorly or not getting enough nutrients. Recognize these habits without putting any blame on yourself. By simply identifying them, you will have a better idea of what needs to change. When you can reevaluate yourself while keeping a neutral mindset, you will be more likely to make productive changes in your life. Acknowledge that you might not have the healthiest coping mechanisms at the moment, but this can change if you truly want it to.

Think about what you truly want for yourself and what you truly want out of your life. Try to think beyond the things that give you instant gratification. This can be a deep realization to come to, so it is important that you do not rush yourself. You can meditate on the idea or write down your thoughts in order to keep them organized. Try to only think about the things that will actually serve your purpose and allow you to meet your goals. By getting rid of the idea that temporary fixes are going to help you, then you will be able to focus on what is really most important. It can be difficult to truly dissect these things, but it is good to have an idea of where you currently are in your life. This is all going to matter as you begin your Keto journey.

Make a pact to get rid of your bad habits and bring in the new habits to take their place. When you have a solution present, it feels less like you are giving up on something and more like you are simply reframing your way of thinking. This is how you are going to keep the optimism flowing freely while you are on the Keto diet. Never take anything away from yourself, food or otherwise, without first thinking of a positive replacement for it. When you do things this way, you will never feel like you are being deprived of the things that you want the most. You will instead be teaching yourself and your body how to desire healthy alternatives.

Food and happiness are closely linked in more ways than you think. Aside from eating foods that comfort you when you are feeling down, there are actually some foods that naturally boost your happiness because they are good for your brain. These foods often fall into the protein category and they work by keeping your brain active and sharp. When you do not exercise your brain, much like any other muscle in your body, it becomes weak and tired. Doing so becomes a hassle because it feels like it is not able to function as it once used to. By eating healthy fats and omega 3 rich proteins on a daily basis, your brain is going to have the fuel to stay active. It will be exercising itself and functioning at its prime. This will keep you happier because you will be aware of exactly what you are doing and feeling.

When you do not have a clear head, life can become complicated. Living with this cloud hovering over you can often feel like something is wrong when everything is actually okay. The brain is very powerful, and it can lead you to many different conclusions if you are not careful. One major factor to look into if you begin to experience depression is your diet. While it might seem trivial, it is a factor in the way that your brain operates. You might be going through a lot of dark, personal issues but that isn't the only problem. If you fill your body with junk food and preservatives, it doesn't get the proper nutrients to produce the right chemicals in your brain that will make you happy. Instead, it will just be running off of sugar until it crashes and then the cycle repeats.

Staying optimistic while on the Keto diet does require some basic knowledge about the brain. A depressed brain is harder to keep happy if you aren't eating food that is packed with nutrients. After your first week full of protein, make note of how your brain feels and how clear your thoughts are. Most likely, you will find that you are able to think much clearer with more confidence. Being able to use your brain in the way that you know you are capable of provides you with a sense of purpose and stability. This is important to any human being because living without a purpose is one way to trigger depression. This can make life feel very overwhelming and scary. Being on Keto is great because you have an automatic purpose. When you feel the benefits of the results in your brain, this is just another positive aspect of the diet making its way into your lifestyle.

Keeping Yourself Inspired

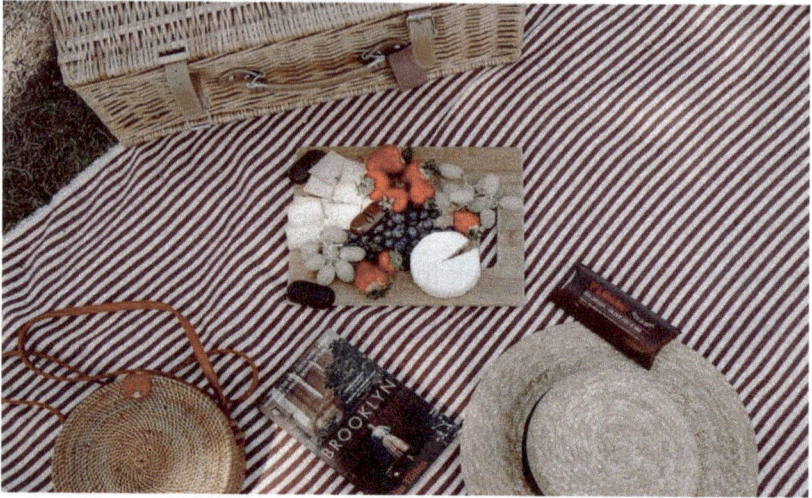

It is important to seek out inspiration with everything that you do in life. Having a source of inspiration will provide you with even more motivation to reach your goals. In a way, this guide can serve as your first source of inspiration as you begin your Keto journey. By reading about the facts and benefits of the lifestyle, you should feel excited and ready to begin. Once you get the hang of Keto, you start to become your own inspiration. You can do so by being persistent with your routine.

Everyone has routines that they follow throughout the day, whether they change frequently or remain the same. Having routines means that you have a sense of stability, which is great! Your routine should be regular enough to keep you on track, yet flexible enough to never become boring or stale. A great routine has room for mistakes and plenty of room for changes, if necessary.

Each morning recite some positive affirmations to yourself as you begin your day. These affirmations can be as simple as "I can do this," or as complex as you want them to be. No matter what is going on in your life, if you start the day with positivity, you are likely going to be able to return to this positivity later on. Use your breakfast time as a chance for you to enjoy the fact that you are nourishing your body. No matter what you are eating, any Keto breakfast is going to prepare you for the day ahead. If you are bringing lunch with you to work, make sure that it is packed and ready to go with you. Without having to struggle to decide what you'd like to eat for lunch that day, you are taking away one stressor. The more stressors that you are able to eliminate, the better your day will go.

Remember to savor your lunch once you get the chance to eat it. Sit down and enjoy your food. Let the quality and healing properties of the food inspire you. Your lunch break should be used for eating and nothing else. If you are multitasking during this time, your body isn't going to reach a state of relaxation. All of the tension and stress that you have been holding onto throughout the morning is going to follow you as you eat your lunch. This can cause your digestive system to act up, potentially even causing you indigestion or an upset stomach. Stress tends to build up in your stomach which can definitely influence your appetite. Know that no matter what is going on around you, you'll be able to return to it after you enjoy your lunch. It's amazing what a few moments of relaxation can do to break up all of the different elements that you have been experiencing throughout your day.

If you do find an opportunity to eat out with your friends, take this as a personal challenge of your knowledge about the Keto diet. Think about any substitutions that can be made to classic restaurant food. Know that you shouldn't be ashamed that you are focused on your health. Being on a diet isn't the end of your fun and happiness. It is meant to become a regular part of your lifestyle. Your friends and loved ones should also be understanding and supportive of your cause. If you show them how the Keto diet is making you feel great, then there is no reason why the ones who care about you most would make you feel guilty for being on the diet. Your support system is very important during this time, so make sure that you are aware of the company that you are keeping. A good support system should be an inspirational, encouraging and supportive voice while you are on your journey. You might even find that they will become interested in trying out the diet for themselves.

As you have been learning about the Keto diet for yourself, it is likely that you have been able to see past many of the stigmas that people talk about. This happens with nearly any diet plan because dieting has been a controversial topic in society for the last several decades. By spreading accurate information about the Keto diet and being a living example of someone who is on it, you are doing your best to educate those around you. When you can show people that you aren't actually "starving" and that you are receiving benefits such as weight loss and energy boosts, this can truly change minds about how the Keto diet really works. People are going to be naturally skeptical, but as long as you stay true to what you know, you will be able to continue seeing the successful results that you desire.

Let dinner time be your chance to explore new options. Whether you are eating in with the family or going out to a new restaurant, try to have something new for dinner each night to keep you intrigued with the diet. There are so many options for what you can make given the ingredients that Keto boosts. You will always have a protein-packed entree that is full of flavor. Because you are able to cook with butter and oil, all of your favorite dishes can be replicated without having to skip over them. People truly enjoy how many of their favorite savory meals are included in the guidelines of the Keto diet. Some people say that it almost feels too good to be true that they are still able to eat these things! Eating healthy, healing foods is definitely a source of inspiration.

When you take the time to make sure that your body feels great by exercising, know that this is a reason to be inspired by yourself and your choices. It can be difficult to get up and moving, especially while on a new diet. Commend yourself for the effort that you put into your workout routines and know that, paired with the Keto diet, you are going to be seeing results very soon. When you get into these habits, you will be more likely to return to them again in the future on your own. They become less like tasks to complete and more like normal parts of your day that you can expect. When you get into the full swing of Keto, it should feel natural and effortless.

Conclusion

Now that you are familiar with the Keto diet on many levels, you should feel confident in your ability to start your own Keto journey. This diet plan isn't going to hinder you or limit you, so do your best to keep this in mind as you begin changing your lifestyle and adjusting your eating habits. Packed with good fats and plenty of protein, your body is going to go through a transformation as it works to see these things as energy. Before you know it, your body will have an automatically accessible reserve that you can utilize at any time. Whether you need a boost of energy first thing in the morning or a second wind to keep you going throughout the day, this will already be inside of you.

As you take care of yourself through the next few years, you can feel great knowing that the Keto diet aligns with the anti-aging lifestyle that you seek. Not only does it keep you looking great and feeling younger, but it also acts as a preventative barrier from various ailments and conditions. The body tends to weaken as you age, but Keto helps to keep a shield up in front of it by giving you plenty of opportunities to burn energy and create muscle mass. Instead of taking the things that you need in order to feel great, Keto only takes what you have in abundance. This is how you will always end up feeling your best each day.

Arguably one of the best diets around, Keto keeps you feeling so great because you have many meal options! There is no shortage of delicious and filling meals that you can eat while you are on any of the Keto diet plans. You can even take this diet with you as you eat out at restaurants and at friends' houses. As long as you can remember the simple guidelines, you should have no problems staying on track with Keto. Cravings become almost non-existent as your body works to change the way it digests. Instead of relying on glucose in your bloodstream, your body switches focus. It begins using fat as soon as you reach the state of ketosis that you are aiming for. The best part is, you do not have to do anything other than eating within your fat/protein/carb percentages. Your body will do the rest on its own.

Because this is a way that your body can properly function for long periods of time, Keto is proven to be more than a simple fad diet. Originating with a medical background for helping epilepsy patients, the Keto diet has been tried and tested for decades. Many successful studies align with the knowledge that Keto really works. Whether you are trying to be on the diet for a month or a year, both are just as healthy for you. Keto is an adjustment, but it is one that will continue benefiting you for as long as you are able to keep it up. If you are ready to feel great and look great from the inside out, you can begin your Keto journey with the confidence that it is truly going to make a difference in your life. The natural signs of aging and hormonal imbalances of being a woman are not enough to hold you back when you are actively participating in a balanced Keto diet.

Change your life today and enjoy the many benefits of a Keto diet.

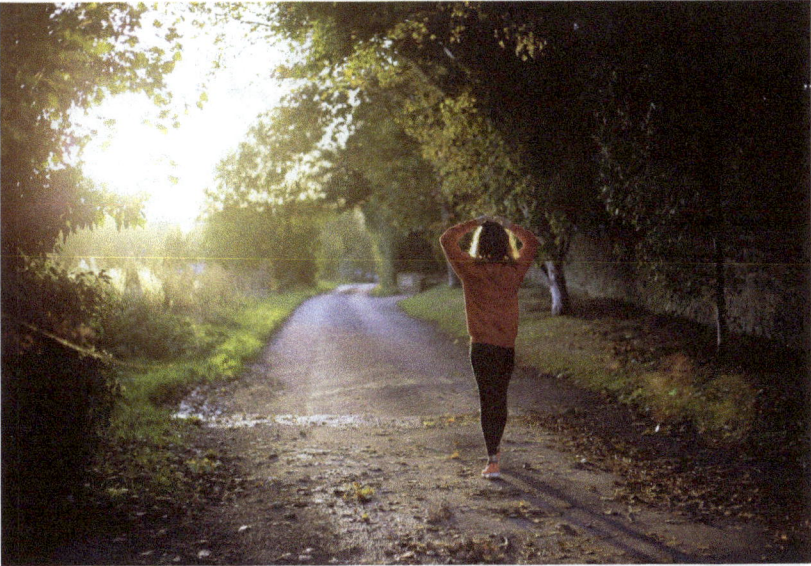

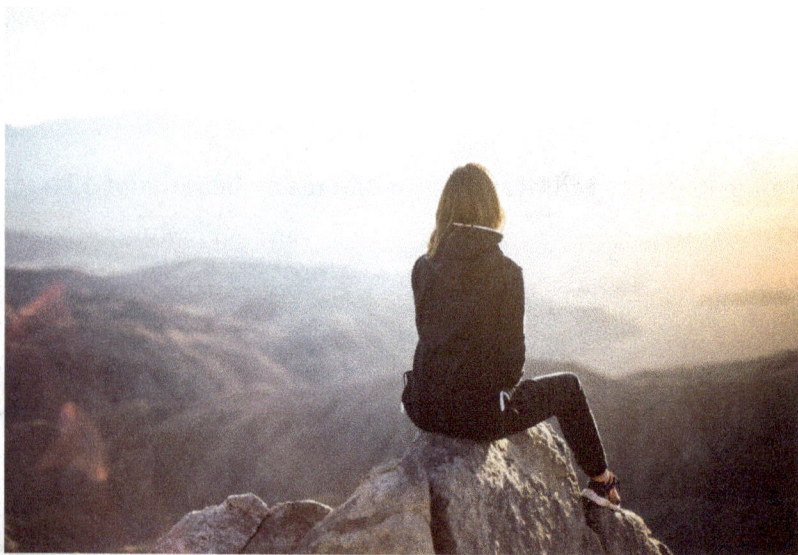

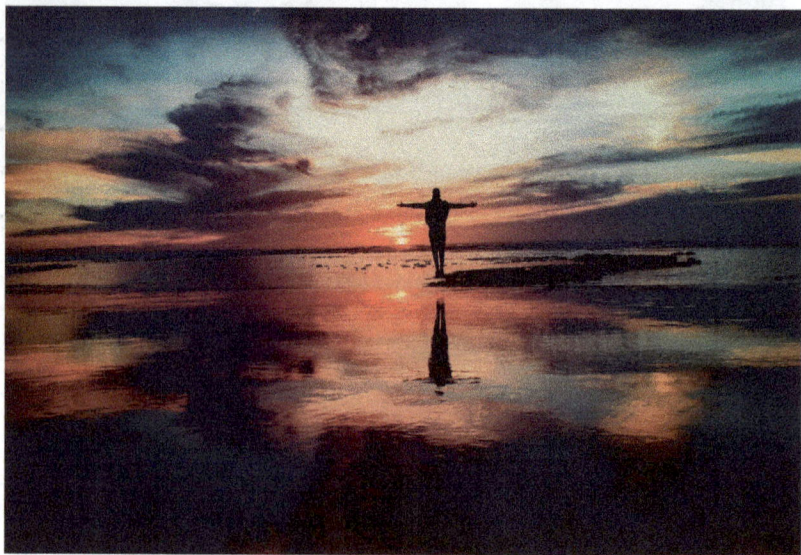

References

Alley Interactive. (2020, January 6). This Anti-Aging Keto Plan Helps You Shed Pounds in a Flash. Retrieved February 4, 2020, from https://www.womansworld.com/posts/diets/anti-aging-keto-172222

Ciccarelli, D. (2019, September 13). Keto Energy: How a Ketogenic Diet is the Secret to Sustained Energy. Retrieved February 4, 2020, from https://perfectketo.com/keto-energy/

Ciccarelli, L. (2019, November 26). Keto For Women: How to Do It Right and Lose Weight. Retrieved February 4, 2020, from https://perfectketo.com/keto-for-women/

Clarke, C. (2019, September 13). Targeted Ketogenic Diet: An In-depth Look. Retrieved February 4, 2020, from https://www.ruled.me/targeted-ketogenic-diet-indepth-look/

Dunn, S. T. (2019, June 3). 10 Reasons to Eat Clean. Retrieved February 4, 2020, from https://www.cleaneatingmag.com/clean-diet/10-reasons-to-eat-clean

Healthy Eating: Changing Your Eating Habits. (2020). Retrieved February 4, 2020, from https://wa.kaiserpermanente.org/kbase/topic.jhtml?docId=ad1169

Hyman, M., MD. (2019, October 21). 7 Reasons You Need to Detox! Retrieved February 4, 2020, from https://drhyman.com/blog/2015/03/12/7-reasons-you-need-to-detox/ Kubala, M. (2018, April 3). The Keto Flu: Symptoms and How to Get Rid of It. Retrieved February 10, 2020, from https://www.healthline.com/nutrition/keto-flu-symptoms#get-rid

Kubala, M. J. S. (2018, October 30). What Is the Cyclical Ketogenic Diet? Everything You Need to Know. Retrieved February 4, 2020, from https://www.healthline.com/nutrition/cyclical-ketogenic-diet#basic-steps

Leonard, J. (2020, January 29). Keto diet: 1-week meal plan and tips. Retrieved February 4, 2020, from https://www.medicalnewstoday.com/articles/327309.php#1-week-sample-meal-plan

Mawer, R. M. (2018, July 30). The Ketogenic Diet: A Detailed Beginner's Guide to Keto. Retrieved February 4, 2020, from https://www.healthline.com/nutrition/ketogenic-diet-101#types

Migala, J. (2019, November 4). The Keto Diet: 7-Day Menu and Comprehensive Food List | Everyday Health. Retrieved February 4, 2020, from https://www.everydayhealth.com/diet-nutrition/ketogenic-diet/comprehensive-ketogenic-diet-food-list-follow/mindbodygreen. (2019, October 24).

Why The Ketogenic Diet Is Great For Hormone Balance. Retrieved February 4, 2020, from https://www.mindbodygreen.com/articles/why-the-ketogenic-diet-is-great-for-hormone-balance

Occhipinti, M., PhD. (2018, September 10). What is the History and Evolution of the Keto Diet? Retrieved February 4, 2020, from https://www.afpafitness.com/blog/what-is-the-history-and-evolution-of-the-keto-diet

Spritzler, R. F. D. (2017, January 23). 16 Foods to Eat on a Ketogenic Diet. Retrieved February 4, 2020, from https://www.healthline.com/nutrition/ketogenic-diet-foods#section1

StockSnap.io - Beautiful Free Stock Photos (CC0). (2020c). Retrieved February 4, 2020, from https://stocksnap.io/

www.ingramcontent.com/pod-product-compliance
Lightning Source LLC
Chambersburg PA
CBHW050217270326
41914CB00003BA/458